A Handbook for Stu[dent] Nurses

Introducing Key Issues Relevant for Practice

Nursing titles from Reflect Press Ltd

Clinical Skills for Student Nurses edited by Robin Richardson
ISBN 978 1 906052 04 1

Understanding Research and Evidence-based Practice by Bruce Lindsay
ISBN 978 1 906052 01 0

Values for Care Practice by Sue Cuthbert and Jan Quallington
ISBN 978 1 906052 05 8

Communication and Interpersonal Skills by Elaine Donnelly and
Lindsey Neville
ISBN 978 1 906052 06 5

Numeracy, Clinical Calculations and Basic Statistics by Neil Davison
ISBN 978 1 906052 07 2

Essential Study Skills edited by Marjorie Lloyd and Peggy Murphy
ISBN 978 1 906052 14 0

Safe and Clean Care by Tina Tilmouth with Simon Tilmouth
ISBN 978 1 906052 08 9

Neonatal Care edited by Amanda Williamson and Kenda Crozier
ISBN 978 1 906052 09 6

Fundamentals of Diagnostic Imaging edited by Anne-Marie Dixon
ISBN 978 1 906052 10 2

Fundamentals of Nursing Care by Anne Llewellyn and Sally Hayes
ISBN 978 1 906052 13 3

The Care and Wellbeing of Older People edited by Angela Kydd, Tim Duffy
and F.J. Raymond Duffy
ISBN 978 1 906052 15 7

Palliative Care edited by Elaine Stevens and Janette Edwards
ISBN 978 1 906052 16 4

Nursing in the UK: A Handbook for Nurses from Overseas
by Wendy Benbow and Gill Jordan
ISBN 978 1 906052 00 3

Interpersonal Skills for the People Professions
edited by Lindsey Neville
ISBN 978 1 906052 18 8

For further details on these and other Reflect Press titles please visit our
website at www.reflectpress.co.uk

A Handbook for Student Nurses

Introducing Key Issues Relevant for Practice

By Wendy Benbow and Gill Jordan

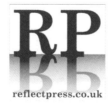

reflectpress.co.uk

First published in 2009

ISBN: 978 1 906052 19 5

British Library Cataloguing in Publication Data
A catalogue record for this book is available from the British Library

The authors and publisher have made every attempt to ensure the content of this
book is up-to-date and accurate. However, healthcare knowledge and information is
changing all the time so the reader is advised to double-check any information in this
text on drug usage, treatment procedures, the use of equipment, etc. to confirm
that it complies with the latest safety recommendations, standards of practice
and legislation, as well as local Trust policies and procedures.

Production project management by Deer Park Productions
Typeset by Kestrel Data, Exeter, Devon
Cover design by Oxmed
Printed and bound in the UK by Bell & Bain Ltd, Glasgow
Distributed by BEBC, Albion Close, Parkstone, Poole, Dorset BH12 3LL

Published by Reflect Press Ltd
11 Attwyll Avenue
Exeter
Devon, EX2 5HN
UK
01392 204400

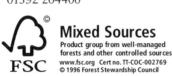

Mixed Sources
Product group from well-managed
forests and other controlled sources
www.fsc.org Cert no. TT-COC-002769
© 1996 Forest Stewardship Council

reflectpress.co.uk

Reflect Press Ltd
www.reflectpress.co.uk

Contents

Introduction

The Nursing and Midwifery Council (NMC) is responsible for setting standards of proficiency that define the overarching principles of being able to practise as a nurse, and they must be achieved before students are eligible to join the register. The aim of this handbook is to highlight and address many of the key issues that surround these standards of proficiency and relate them to the context of the practice setting.

This handbook has been written primarily for student nurses, whether undertaking a diploma, advanced diploma or degree along with their professional qualification; but it is envisaged that students undertaking further education access courses and Level 3 NVQ (health care) will also find the information helpful. The content is also relevant for health care assistants and assistant practitioners. The information within the book is relevant to all areas of nursing, and all branches of nursing.

A Handbook for Student Nurses is designed so that you can utilise individual chapters as a quick source of reference although, along with the activities and further reading, it may serve as a starting point for more in-depth study. Where websites are identified, these are only suggested sources of further information and others may be found through general search engines such as **www.google.co.uk**. Although the emphasis is mainly related to health care in England, we do refer to Scotland, Wales and Northern Ireland when appropriate.

AUTHOR BIOGRAPHIES

Wendy Benbow

Following qualification as a registered nurse in 1969, Wendy worked for two years in genito-urinary surgery and major spinal injuries before moving into community nursing. Over a 14-year period Wendy was involved in a variety of roles that included community nursing sister, practice work teacher and nurse manager, as well as time seconded for research and co-ordinating pre-registration student placements for the local acute hospital.

After a year out to complete her teaching qualification, Wendy moved into full-time education in 1985. Since then, she has been involved in both teaching on and managing a range of pre- and post-registration courses, programme development, regionally funded research and national project development. She is currently working as an associate lecturer for the Open University.

Gill Jordan

On qualifying as a registered nurse in 1978, Gill completed her Orthopaedic Nursing Certificate and moved to New Zealand where she worked in a large orthopaedic teaching hospital, ultimately as a ward sister of a trauma orthopaedic ward.

On her return to the UK in 1988, Gill moved into nurse education. Since then, she has been involved in a variety of courses and professional development programmes, both as a teacher and programme leader. These have included courses leading to professional registration, Return to Practice, Overseas Nurses Programme, conversion courses and various post-registration undergraduate programmes.

Chapter 1

Nurse Education and Mentorship

This chapter provides an overview of the preparation nurses undertake during their pre-registration programmes, and an insight into the registered nurse's role in supporting students.

Outcomes

On completion of this chapter you should:

- have an outline view of programmes leading to nurse registration;

- understand the need for mentorship in nursing;

- be able to define the qualities required to be a good mentor.

NURSE EDUCATION

Background

Nurse education, prior to the 1990s, was a traditional 'apprentice' style training, where nurses were based in a school of nursing within the hospital where they carried out their clinical work. There were then two levels of nurse qualification – Registered Nurse (1ˢᵗ level nurse) and Enrolled Nurse (2ⁿᵈ level nurse), the former being a three-year training programme, and the latter a more practically based two-year training programme. However, in the 1980s, there was a push towards establishing nursing in a 'more professional light', and a recognition that nurses were taking on work more traditionally carried out by doctors, while health care assistants were undertaking work that had been carried out by registered nurses. This was coupled with the appreciation that there

1

were common elements that underpinned all nursing practice whichever 'branch' (mental health, learning disability, adult, child health) of nursing was studied (RCN, 2004).

The 1990s saw the advent of 'Project 2000' – a new style of nurse training that transformed pre-registration nurse education at the time and continues to do so. As you know, nurses now study in universities (higher education institutes) and exit their programme not only with a first-level professional nursing qualification (RN), but also with a higher-educational qualification.

NURSE EDUCATION TODAY

The NMC sets the standards of education and training for pre-registration nursing programmes (Nursing and Midwifery Order, 2001). They determine the level of entry and content of programmes, and universities have to have validation and regular reviews from them to run their programmes. Along with NMC standards, universities also have to comply with standards set by the Quality Assurance Agency (QAA) – these being general standards for all courses run within higher education. At present students normally complete pre-registration nursing programmes in three years of full-time study. They are offered at diploma, advanced diploma or degree level; the level the student studies at usually being dependent on their academic qualifications on leaving school. However, the NMC (2008) is currently reviewing the minimum academic award for students exiting a pre-registration programme, and it is highly likely that in the future this will be at degree level only.

Whatever the level of your study, 50 per cent of time is spent on theoretical aspects of nursing and 50 per cent in practice areas – this currently equates to 2300 hours each of practice and theory. At all academic levels you have to complete a common foundation programme within your first year where aspects of nursing common to all areas of practice are studied. Then, if you have achieved the required NMC competencies for the first year, you specialise for the remaining two years in the branches of adult, child, mental health or learning disabilities nursing. Although you should identify which branch of nursing you wish to ultimately register in on commencement of your programme, most universities allow transfer to a different branch at the end of the first year. Likewise, if you excel on a diploma or advanced diploma programme, most universities allow you to transfer to a degree programme, or vice versa if the level of study proves too challenging for a student initially enrolled on the degree programme.

Clinical practice placements are an essential and integral part of the programme and enable you to experience a range of clinical environments each year. During your practice hours you are deemed supernumerary and are not included in the number of staff in the clinical placement. You are assessed in practice by a mentor via a set of competencies issued by the NMC (a series of standards that students have to achieve both during and at the end of your three-year programme). The competencies fall into four domains of practice, which are:

- professional and ethical practice;
- care delivery;
- care management;
- personal and professional development.

(NMC, 2004a)

Standards of proficiency for nursing (NMC, 2004a, p. 5)

The NMC has to be satisfied that its standards for granting a person a licence to practice are being met as required, and in accordance with the law. It does this by setting standards that must be achieved in order to maintain public confidence, and therefore protecting the public (Peate, 2006). These standards must be achieved before you are eligible to join the register and are outlined below:

- Manage oneself, one's practice, and that of others, in accordance with *The Code: Standards of conduct, performance and ethics for nurses and midwives* (the Code), recognising one's own abilities and limitations.
- Practise in accordance within an ethical and legal framework which ensures the primacy of patient and client interest and well-being and respects confidentiality.
- Practise in a fair and anti-discriminatory way, acknowledging the differences in beliefs and cultural practices of individuals or groups.
- Engage in, develop and disengage from therapeutic relationships through the use of appropriate communication and interpersonal skills.
- Create and utilise opportunities to promote the health and well-being of patients, clients and groups.
- Undertake and document a comprehensive, systematic and accurate nursing assessment of the physical, psychological, social and spiritual needs of patients, clients and communities.
- Formulate and document a plan of nursing care, where possible in partnership with patients, clients, their carers and family and friends, within a framework of informed consent.

- Based on the best available evidence, apply knowledge and an appropriate repertoire of skills indicative of safe nursing practice.
- Provide a rationale for the nursing care delivered which takes account of social, cultural, spiritual, legal, political and economic influences.
- Evaluate and document the outcomes of nursing and other interventions.
- Demonstrate sound clinical judgement across a range of differing professional and care delivery contexts.
- Contribute to public protection by creating and maintaining a safe environment of care through the use of quality assurance and risk-management strategies.
- Demonstrate knowledge of effective inter-professional working practices which respect and utilise the contributions of members of the health and social care team.
- Delegate duties to others, as appropriate, ensuring that they are supervised and monitored.
- Demonstrate key skills.
- Demonstrate a commitment to the need for continuing professional development and personal supervision activities in order to enhance knowledge, skills, values and attitudes needed for safe and effective nursing practice.
- Enhance the professional development and safe practice of others through peer support, leadership, supervision and teaching.

To support these standards, and to focus education and clinical experience on key aspects that the NMC has identified as areas of concern relating to skills deficit at entry to branch level and at the point of registration, the NMC introduced *Essential Skills Clusters* into the standards in 2007. These are generic skills statements, applicable to all branches of nursing and all fields of practice, set out under the broad headings of:

- care and compassion;
- communication;
- organisational aspects of care;
- infection prevention and control;
- nutrition and fluid maintenance;
- medicines management.

These skills are specifically tested by the university in the same way that existing competencies are tested.

Further information

If you wish to know more about pre-registration nursing programmes there is an excellent section on the Practice Based Learning website **www.practicebasedlearning.org** (click on 'Case Studies' then click on 'Nursing Case Study') that discusses practice education in nursing and includes topics such as the pre-registration nursing courses and mentorship. Alternatively visit the NMC website – **www.nmc-uk.org**

The title 'Registered Nurse' is protected in law and can only be used by someone registered with the NMC. At the end of your training, your course director will complete a declaration of good health and good character on your behalf which must be received by the NMC before it can register you (see Chapter 4 on 'Legal and professional issues'). Once registered you are accountable to the NMC and have to abide by their standards and guidelines, most importantly *The Code: Standards of conduct, performance and ethics for nurses and midwives* (2008).

CLINICAL PRACTICE PLACEMENTS

Practice placements are an essential and integral part of a nurse education programme. They provide unique learning experiences and opportunities for you as a student and enable you to develop professional competencies that cannot be readily acquired elsewhere, but they need to be planned, structured, managed and co-ordinated (ENB/DH, 2001). Stuart (2003) believes that your clinical experience should be much more than just learning what to do and how to do it – it should be about the education of students who will one day be professional peers, colleagues and co-learners.

The NMC, in reflecting European Union requirements (EEC/89/595), stipulates that your practice experience must include direct contact with healthy and/or sick individuals, and must enable you to meet all your relevant statutory requirements. All your hours must be verified and you must complete a three-month placement at the end of your third year. The nature of your placements has to be extensive in order to provide learning opportunities that reflect the large range of health care needs experienced by the population, but the timing, length and type of placement will differ between individual universities (**www. practicebasedlearning.org**). Although you are 'supernumerary', you are generally expected to complete the same shift patterns as your mentor, and to gain experience of night working.

The Royal College of Nursing (RCN) (2002, p. 2) lists 15 points they believe are important for your learning in an effective practice placement. Placements should help you to:

- meet the statutory and regulatory requirements and, where applicable, European directives;
- achieve the required learning outcomes and competencies according to regulatory body requirements for pre-registration education (NMC, 2004a);
- recognise the diversity of learning opportunities available within health and social care environments;
- work within a wide range of rapidly changing health and social services that recognise the continuing nature of care;
- provide the full range of nursing care to patients;
- demonstrate an appreciation of the unpredictable and dynamic nature of the clinical setting as a learning environment within a multi-professional approach to care;
- feel valued and safe within a culture that recognises the importance of adult learning;
- maintain your supernumerary status;
- work alongside mentors who are appropriately prepared, creating a partnership with them;
- identify appropriate learning opportunities to meet your learning needs, linking general learning objectives to specific experiences within the practice context;
- use time effectively, creating opportunities to enable the application of theory to practice and vice versa;
- apply knowledge gained in the use of experiential and enquiry- or problem-based learning, within the practice context;
- reflect contemporary thinking within modern health care to evaluate the effectiveness of care provided, and, based on research evidence, continue to develop your competence in both interpersonal and practical skills;
- give an honest, evaluative feedback of your practice experiences to aid the audit process for the practice placement;
- develop skills in information technology to access information within the placement area.

> **Activity**
>
> The RCN published *Helping Students Get the Best from their Practice Placement* in 2002, which is an excellent document – try to get a copy of this and read through it.

The role of the mentor

Many practice-based professions, including nursing, traditionally rely on clinical staff to support, supervise and teach students in practice settings – the underlying rationale being that in working alongside practitioners, students will learn from experts in a safe, supportive and educationally adjusted environment (Benner, 1984).

The form of support afforded to students can be difficult to define. Within nursing the term 'mentor' is generally used to describe a person who supports and assesses student nurses, while the term 'preceptor' is used for a supporter of a post-registration nurse during their first few months post qualifying. The most popular definition of a mentor comes from the document *Preparation for Mentors and Teachers* (ENB/Department of Health, 2001, p. 6), which states 'a mentor is a nurse who facilitates learning and supervises and assesses students in the practice setting'. The NMC states that all students on pre-registration nursing education programmes must be supported and assessed by qualified mentors (NMC, 2006a).

Mentors are expected to have the skills to enable you to undergo appropriate and valuable learning experiences and to assess your competence. They must have the equivalent of one year's full-time post-registration experience, be on the same part of the register as you aspire to, and have undertaken specific preparation for the role comprising a mentorship course accredited by a higher education institution. The content of such a mentorship course must include (NMC, 2006a, p. 6):

- establishing effective working relationships;
- facilitation of learning;
- assessment and accountability;
- evaluation of learning;
- creating an environment for learning;
- context of practice;
- evidence-based practice;
- leadership.

In August 2006 the NMC issued its document *Standards to Support Learning and Assessment in Practice* (NMC, 2006a), which reiterated the need for all students to have mentors but also introduced the role of a 'sign-off' mentor. The sign-off mentor must have undergone a mentor preparation course and met additional specific criteria. The sign-off mentor is responsible (and accountable) for signing off a student at the end of their training period, confirming they have achieved all your competencies, are fit for practice and have the necessary knowledge, skills and competence to take on the role of a registered nurse.

Nevertheless, despite this NMC standard, there is an expectation and requirement that all registered nurses play a key part in the preparation of students for registration. This was emphasised explicitly in the 2004 version of *The Code of Professional Conduct* (NMC, 2004b, clause 6.4), but the new code simply states that registered nurses must be willing to share their skills and experience for the benefit of their colleagues (NMC, 2008). However, the Department of Health (1999) still maintains that every practitioner shares the responsibility to support and teach the next generation of nurses, and that it is important that nurses are taught by those with practical and recent experience of nursing.

Activity

Take a few minutes to answer the following questions.
- What qualities would you like to see in your mentor?
- Can you think of any obstacles to being effectively mentored?
- What are the benefits to you as a student in having a mentor?

The RCN (2007, p. 5) states that mentors are required to offer you support and guidance, and to help you make sense of your practice through:

- the application of theory;
- assessing, evaluating and giving constructive feedback;
- facilitating reflection on practice, performance and experiences.

And furthermore that a mentor should:

- be a positive role model;
- be knowledgeable and skilled;
- help you develop skills and confidence;
- promote a professional relationship with you;

- provide you with the appropriate level of supervision;
- assist with planned learning experiences;
- offer honest and constructive feedback.

However, it is not only your mentor who has responsibilities. You also have a responsibility to (RCN, 2002):

- be proactive in seeking out experiences for your level of practice and competence with the support of your mentor;
- demonstrate a willingness to work as part of the team in the delivery of safe patient care;
- learn to express your needs and adopt a questioning, reflective approach to your learning within the multidisciplinary team;
- use your mentor for guidance and support to enable you to achieve your learning outcomes and satisfactorily complete your practice assessments;
- seek help from appropriate clinical managers or link lecturers if the mentor relationship is not working, to enable the achievement of the learning outcomes;
- ensure that clinical skills required at each stage in the programme are attempted under the supervision of a skilled practitioner, with comments provided by both you and your mentor;
- utilise learning opportunities outside the practice placements and, where possible, work with specialist practitioners;
- identify the role of professionals within other contexts of the organisation or community, for example, in X-ray, pharmacy and outpatients;
- give and receive constructive feedback;
- reflect on your progress to increase self-awareness, confidence and competence.

Also (RCN, 2007):

- read your higher education institution's (HEI's) charter and student handbooks;
- familiarise yourself with handbooks related to your specific programme (these will include assessment of practice documentation);
- recognise the purpose of your placement experience and ensure you are clear about the expectations of the placement provider;
- ensure you have some theoretical knowledge relating to the placement;
- contact your placement and mentor prior to starting;
- highlight any support needs to your mentor;

- act professionally with regard to punctuality, attitude and image, and dress according to uniform policy;
- maintain confidentiality;
- maintain effective communication with patients, mentors, and link personnel from both the placement and HEI;
- adhere to the NMC *Guide for Students of Nursing and Midwifery* (2005a):
  - understand your responsibility and accountability, always work under the supervision of a registered nurse;
  - respect the wishes of patients at all times;
  - identify yourself as a student to the patient at the first opportunity;
  - uphold patient confidentiality in accordance with the NMC's *Code* (2008);
  - do not participate in procedures for which you have not been fully prepared or in which you are not adequately supervised.

As previously stated, one of the major roles of the mentor is to assess you on your clinical practice. All mentors can assess specific competencies and confirm their achievement, but only sign-off mentors can confirm overall achievement of proficiency and therefore fitness for entry to the register. Your consistency of performance is measured via continuous assessment which is, in the most part, by your mentor directly observing the care that you deliver. This is recorded within your 'Ongoing Achievement of Practice Record' which it is your responsibility to take from placement to placement.

Further Information

Along with *Helping Students get the Best from their Practice Placement* (2002) the RCN also publishes a booklet *Guidance for Mentors of Nursing Students and Midwifery* (2007), which you may find helpful.

PRECEPTORSHIP

There is a general acknowledgement that all professions need a period of preceptorship following qualification for professional registration, and this of course includes nursing. The UKCC (now NMC) report *Fitness for Practice* published in 1999 highlighted this in saying: 'All newly-qualified registrants should receive a properly supported period of induction and preceptorship when they begin their employment.' The UKCC further added that the health care professions should actively be encouraged to learn with and from one another, which is reflected in the increasing number of preceptorship programmes available.

Preceptorship comes under the banner of 'lifelong learning' and the NMC has republished its document *Supporting Nurses and Midwives Through Lifelong Learning* (2005b). In this document the NMC believes that all newly-registered nurses and midwives should have a formal period of support under the guidance of a preceptor. The precise length of time will vary according to individual need and local circumstances, but the NMC (2006b) believes that four months is a suitable time. In many ways, every time a newly qualified nurse works alongside more experienced professional colleagues, they can learn from their colleagues and be guided by them as the newly qualified nurse further develops their own skills and confidence.

Formal preceptorship, however, means that the newly registered nurse is allocated a named individual, working in the same area of practice, who is on hand to guide, help, advise and support. The NMC states (2005b, p. 1) that: 'this doesn't mean that they accompany the newly registered nurse everywhere they go and constantly look over their shoulder, but it does mean they can be called if help is needed with a procedure or a situation not encountered before; or if they simply feel that they need support and guidance'.

Preceptors, like mentors, should be first-level registered nurses who have had at least 12 months' experience as a registered nurse and understand the concept of preceptorship. There are no formal qualifications to be a preceptor, but preceptors must (NMC, 2006b, p. 1):

- know about the newly registered nurse's training and experience and be able to identify learning needs;
- help the newly registered nurse apply knowledge to practice;
- be able to act as a resource to facilitate the newly qualified nurse's professional development.

Preceptorship is not a mandatory requirement and the NMC has no power to enforce the system, but most NHS Trusts run preceptorship courses within their organisations. Some courses are affiliated to universities and nurses can gain academic credit for successfully completing the scheme of study. It is envisaged that all newly qualified staff complete any preceptorship course within one year of qualifying, and that the majority of content will be practice-based.

REFERENCES

Benner, P. (1984) *From Novice to Expert.* California: Addison-Wesley

Department of Health (1999) *Making a Difference. Strengthening the nursing, midwifery and health visiting contribution to health and healthcare.* London: HMSO

English National Board/Department of Health (2001) *Preparation of Mentors and Teachers – A New Framework Guidance.* London: ENB/Department of Health

Nursing and Midwifery Council (2004a) *Standards of Proficiency for Pre-Registration Nursing Education.* London: NMC

Nursing and Midwifery Council (2004b) *Code of Professional Conduct: Standards for conduct, performance and* ethics. London: NMC

Nursing and Midwifery Council (2005a) *An NMC Guide for Students of Nursing and Midwifery.* London: NMC

Nursing and Midwifery Council (2005b) *Supporting Nurses and Midwives through Lifelong Learning.* London: NMC

Nursing and Midwifery Council (2006a) *Standards to Support Learning and Assessment in Practice.* London: NMC

Nursing and Midwifery Council (2006b) *Preceptorship Guidelines,* 21/2006. London: NMC

Nursing and Midwifery Council (2007) *Guidance for the Introduction of the Essential Skills Clusters For Pre-Registration Nursing Programme.* London: NMC

Nursing and Midwifery Council (2008) *The Code: Standards of conduct, performance and ethics for nurses and midwives.* London: NMC

Peate, I. (2006) *Becoming A Nurse in the 21ˢᵗ Century.* Chichester: Wiley

Royal College of Nursing (2002) *Helping Students Get the Best from their Practice Placement.* London: RCN

Royal College of Nursing (2004) *The future nurse: The future for nurse education.* London: RCN

Royal College of Nursing (2007) *Guidance for Mentors of Nursing Students and Midwives.* London: RCN

Stuart, C. (2003) *Assessment, Supervision and Support in Clinical Practice.* New York: Churchill Livingstone

UKCC (1999) *Fitness for Practice.* London: UKCC

Useful websites

www.nmc-uk.org
www.practicebasedlearning.org/home.htm
www.learning-styles-online.com

Chapter 2

Communication

The aim of this chapter is to briefly review the concept of communication in the context of health care delivery.

Outcomes

On completion of this chapter you should have:

- briefly reviewed definitions and the process of communication;
- identified the barriers that may prevent effective communication taking place;
- assessed the skills required for effective and active listening;
- briefly explored the concept of emotional quotient/intelligence.

INTRODUCTION

As a student nurse you will be required to develop and maintain a high level of intra- and interpersonal communication. In fact it is probably one of the most important skills you will need, wherever your area of practice might be, for, to provide competent nursing care, you must be able to communicate effectively. Despite such an importance it is well recognised that many practitioners do not always communicate with others as well as they should.

COMMUNICATION DEFINED

A considerable number of definitions of communication can be found in the literature; here are just a few.

- The exchange of information between two points (**www.micro2000uk.co.uk**).
- The process by which we understand others and in turn endeavour to be understood by them (Burnard, 1997).
- Communication focuses on how people use messages to generate meaning within and across all kinds of contexts, cultures, channels and media (**www.natcom.org**).
- A process by which we assign meaning in an attempt to create shared understanding. This process requires a vast repertoire of intrapersonal/interpersonal processing, listening, observing, speaking, questioning, analysing and evaluating (Bergeson, 2006).

THE COMMUNICATION PROCESS

One way of beginning to explain how communication occurs is the baseline process model of communication (see Figure 1). Based on the work of Shannon and Weaver (1949), this model is still one of the most widely used as a starting point to understand the process of communication.

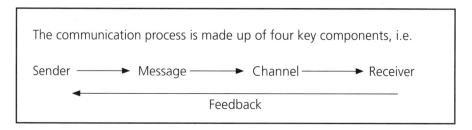

Figure 1 A process model of communication

The sender (transmitter)

The sender is an individual, group or organisation that initiates the communication. All communication begins with the sender and the source is initially responsible for the success of the message. The first step for the sender involves the encoding process.

The message

In order to convey meaning the sender must translate (encode) information into a message in the form of symbols that represent ideas, concepts, etc. These symbols can take on numerous forms such as languages, words or gestures. It is obviously important for the sender to use symbols that are familiar to and appropriate for the intended receiver.

The channel

The channel is the means by which the sender conveys the message. Channels or types of communication generally come under the main headings:

- verbal;
- non-verbal;
- tactile;
- written.

The receiver

After the appropriate channel or channels have been selected, the message enters the decoding stage of the communication process. Decoding is conducted by the receiver. Once the message is received, the stimulus is sent to the brain for interpreting in order to assign some type of meaning, so the receiver is translating the message into their own set of experiences in order to make the symbols meaningful. All interpretations by the receiver are influenced by their experiences, attitudes, knowledge, skills, perceptions and culture (as with the sender's encoding) (Sherman, 1994; Reynolds, 1997; Foulger, 2004).

Although, according to this model, communication is seemingly a simple activity, in essence it is not. It is a complex process in which many other factors need to be considered for effective communication to take place.

INTERPERSONAL SKILLS

Simply put, interpersonal skills are the skills we use to interact or deal with others. Allender and Spradley (2005) suggest that in nursing there are three particular types of interpersonal skills that build on sending and receiving skills and these are:

- respect;
- rapport;
- trust.

Respect

According to Peate (2006, p. 130), respect relates to the ability of a nurse to demonstrate a sincere interest in the patient and his/her needs.

Expressing a genuine wish to understand, show kindness, patience and be concerned for any fears or discomfort the patient may have are also ways of demonstrating respect to the patient and their family.

Rapport

Rapport links to showing respect and is about sympathetic and harmonious relationships, especially ones of emotional affinity and mutual trust.

Trust

Trust is about integrity and having faith and confidence in another. In nursing, Allender and Spradley (2005) suggest trust is developed by providing an open, honest and patient-focused approach.

A further interpersonal skill that it is important to mention here is that of empathy.

Empathy

Definitions of empathy are many but essentially it is about the attempt to understand and share, in a non-judgemental way, the feelings, experiences and concerns of others. Empathy for the most part is a learnt skill or attitude and although it is unlikely that a person who develops such a skill will, or ever could, know exactly what another person actually feels, it is important that the nurse should learn to make the attempt to do so. Empathising with a patient, carer, etc., can only enhance the ability to communicate effectively (**www.scips.worcs.ac.uk**).

Activity

Take a few minutes to reflect back on one or two experiences of being involved in caring for someone where you have utilised the four interpersonal skills identified above.

EMOTIONAL INTELLIGENCE

A relatively recent behavioural model linked to communication and interpersonal skills is that of Emotional Intelligence (EI). Emotional intelligence describes an ability to perceive, assess and manage the emotions of one's self and others (**www.ihhp.com**).

The EI concept suggests that IQ (intelligence quotient), the traditional measure of intelligence, is too limiting as it ignores essential behavioural and character elements. Success in life requires that there are wider areas of EI that dictate and contribute to how successful an individual is. An example often used is that of a person who can be academically brilliant and yet socially and interpersonally inept; we know that despite their possessing a high IQ rating, success does not automatically follow. Essentially EI has two main aspects, namely:

- understanding yourself;
- understanding others and their feelings.

Within these aspects there are four key dimensions.

- **Self-awareness** – knowing one's internal states, preferences, goals, intentions, etc.
- **Social awareness** – awareness of others' feelings, needs and concerns.
- **Self-management** – managing one's internal states, impulses and resources to facilitate reaching goals.
- **Social skills** – adeptness at inducing desirable responses in others.

Extensive research on the subject appears to suggest that the process and outcomes of EI development contain many elements known to reduce stress for individuals and organisations, by decreasing conflict and improving relationships and understanding. Also those who exhibit a high degree of EI tend to be more fulfilled and productive than others in every area of their lives: personal, professional and family.

(www.corporateperspectives.com; www.californiatomorrow.org; www.businessballs.com)

Activity/Further Reading

There is a considerable amount of information on the internet with regard to EI. This includes many sites that provide an opportunity to measure your own level of EI. As a starting point just use a general search engine such as Google.

NON-VERBAL INTERACTION

Verbal and non-verbal skills are closely interrelated and thus non-verbal interaction in health care is also extremely important. Faulkner (1992, p. 76) suggests that, generally, if concurrent verbal and non-verbal messages do not match, then the non-verbal message is the one more likely to be believed. Non-verbal interaction includes the following.

- Body language – which can include:
  - **gesture** – e.g. with hands, arms, head. The gestures people use convey meanings, for example: arms firmly crossed and head turned away can give a negative message to the receiver.
  - **posture** – e.g. sit, stand, slouch. The way that we stand or sit gives information about how we are feeling, for example a nurse sitting slumped in a chair can also give a negative message.
  - **facial expressions** – our faces can show many of our feelings. For example, a frown or a smile shows a very clear message depending on how and when it is used.
  - **eye contact** – maintaining appropriate eye contact when speaking with others helps positive communication. Avoiding eye contact may suggest that you do not really want to communicate, or that you may be telling a lie. Although eye contact for several seconds is good, be careful not to stare or use excessive eye contact as this may make a person feel uncomfortable.
  - **proximity** – most people feel uncomfortable when somebody stands or sits either too close or too far away from them. When this situation happens, it can make communication more difficult.

There is no doubt that when you focus on combining verbal and non-verbal messages in the most effective way possible you should significantly improve your overall communication skills.

Activity

The next time you interact with a patient, carer, etc. stop and think about your non-verbal communication – what message/s do you think you are conveying to the receiver of your message?

BARRIERS TO EFFECTIVE COMMUNICATION

Unfortunately there are many ways in which the message being transmitted in the communication process either never reaches, fails to be understood or is misinterpreted by the receiver. Such barriers to effective communication include the following:

- Non-verbal:
  - negative messages from body language.
- Linguistic:
  - speaking too fast or too slow;
  - too much or too little information given at one time;
  - language differences;
  - regional or national accents;
  - use of technical jargon;
  - restricted or elaborated code of speech;
  - level of voice;
  - tone of voice.
- Cultural:
  - different values, social norms, rules and rituals (relates to both verbal and non-verbal communication), can include social class;
  - perceptions and prejudices.
- Social:
  - background and education;
  - status of the sender – communication is easier if perceived power differential is low.
- Individual/personal:
  - emotional state of the receiver;
  - sensory deficits;
  - poor cognitive skills;
  - fatigue;
  - mistrust;
  - past experiences;
  - need to know – is the information being received important to the receiver or not?
- External/structural:
  - appropriate place for communication (e.g. privacy required);
  - noise;
  - distractions.

Activity

Note down a few key points that you think may help overcome some of the barriers to effective communication listed above.

Overcoming communication barriers

The following are a few points to consider when communicating with service users and their families.

- Select the best location – communicate somewhere that will encourage effective communication.
- Being positive and supportive rather than negative and defensive helps make communication more effective.
- Ensure the best channel for communication has been chosen.
- Be respectful and empathise if appropriate.
- Always be culturally and socially aware with regard to those with whom you are communicating.
- Ensure communication is clear, concise, concrete, correct and courteous.
- Use repetition – repeating messages sometimes using different examples or channels can help the receiver to understand the message being sent.
- Check written communication for spelling errors and ensure the sentences are clear, concise and not ambiguous.
- Develop good listening skills.
  (Burnard, 1992; Adams, 2007; Peate, 2006; **www.witold.me.uk**; **www.scribd.com**)

LISTENING SKILLS

In health care listening is an integral and important part of the communication process. However, it can also be one of the most challenging skills for the nurse to develop. The following can be barriers to effective listening.

- Verbal activities, e.g.:
  - interrupting;
  - asking questions at inappropriate times;
  - preoccupation with other issues;

- perceived time restriction;
- noise;
- individual bias and prejudices;
- hearing only what you want to hear;
- trying to work out what the speaker means rather than listening to what is actually being said.
- Non-verbal activities, e.g.:
  - avoiding eye contact;
  - bored expression, yawning;
  - fiddling and fidgeting;
  - checking watches;
  - tidying papers, etc.;
  - inattention generally.

Unfortunately, some of the above activities happen far too frequently in the busy area of health care practice.

Good listening skills

Good listening skills are not just about being silent and passively receiving the thoughts and feelings of others. To be an effective listener, you need to respond with verbal and non-verbal cues that communicate to the speaker that you are listening to what they are saying. Good listening skills include:

- Give the speaker your undivided attention and look at the speaker directly (not at what else is going on around you).
- Make sure your mind is focused, too. It can be easy to let your mind wander. If you feel your mind wandering, change the position of your body and try to concentrate on the speaker's words.
- Listen for main ideas. Pay special attention to statements that begin with phrases such as 'My point is . . .' or 'The thing to remember is . . .' Also 'listen' to the speaker's non-verbal cues.
- Show you are listening – use body language to convey your attention. For example, nod occasionally, smile and use facial expressions, ensure your posture is open and welcoming.
- Don't interrupt; let the speaker finish before you begin to talk and let yourself finish listening before you begin to speak. Wait for the right opportunity to ask questions.
- If you are not sure you understand what the speaker has said, you need to check this out with them to ensure your understanding is correct. This may be achieved by repeating their words (the last few words of the sentence) or reflecting back in your own words (paraphrasing) what the speaker has said.

- Keep an open and receptive mind to people and their thoughts.
- Be respectful and courteous at all times.

Remember that listening takes time or, more accurately, that you have to take time to listen (Peate, 2006; **www.mindtools.com**; **www.infoplease.com**).

Further reading

Donnelly, E. and Neville, L. (2008) *Health and Social Care Knowledge and Skills: Communication and interpersonal skills*. Exeter: Reflect Press, provides an opportunity to explore further the theory that underpins communication studies and also provides the opportunity to self-assess your own communication and interpersonal skills.

Burnard, P. and Gill, P. (2008) *Culture, Communication and Nursing: A multicultural guide*, explores the wider issues associated with culture and communication in more depth.

REFERENCES

Adams, R. (ed.) (2007) *Foundations in Health and Social Care*. Hampshire: Palgrave Macmillian

Allender, J.A. and Spradley, W. (2005) *Community Health Nursing: Promoting and protecting the public's health* (6th edn). Philadelphia: Lippincott

Bergeson, T. (2006) *Communication*. Available at **www.K12.wa.us/ curriculumstruct/communications/default.aspx** (accessed 9/3/09)

Burnard, P. (1997) *Effective Communication Skills for Health Professionals* (2nd edn). London: Chapman Hall

Faulkner, A. (1992) *Effective Interaction with Patients*. Edinburgh: Churchill Livingstone

Foulger, D. (2004) *Models of the Communication Process*. Available at **http://foulger.info/davis/research/unifiedModelsofCommunication. htm** (accessed 14/4/09)

Micro2000 (2006) *Communication*. Available at **www.micro2000uk. co.uk/hardware_glossary.htm** (accessed 9/3/09)

Peate, I. (2006) *Becoming a Nurse in the 21st Century*. West Sussex: John Wiley and Sons

Reynolds, K. (1997) *What is the transmission of interpersonal communication and what is wrong with it?* Available at **www.aber.ac.uk/media/students/kjr9601.htm** (accessed 14/4/09)

Shannon, C.E. and Weaver, W. (1949) *A Mathematical Model of Communication.* Urbana: University of Illinois Press

Sherman, K.M. (1994) *Communication and Image in Nursing.* Delmar: New York

Useful websites

www.businessballs.com/eq.htm (accessed 16/4/09)

www.californiatomorrow.org/ibe_toolkit/downloads/3_working_tools/2_ebcf/1_hometeam/6_EdPorter_Emotonalintel.pdf (accessed 16/4/09)

www.corporateperspective.com/emot.html (accessed 16/4/09)

www.ihhp.com/what_is_eq.htm (accessed 16/4/09)

www.natcom.org/index.asp?bid=1339 (accessed 14/4/09)

www.scips.worcs.ac.uk/subjects_and_challenges/nursing/nursing_empathy.htm (accessed 15/4/09)

www.witold.me.uk/communication.htm (accessed 15/4/09)

www.scribd.com/doc/10868863/Barriers-to-Communication (accessed 15/4/09)

www.mindtools.com/commsk11/ActiveListening.htm (accessed 15/4/09)

www.infoplease.com/homework/Listeningskills.1.html (accessed 15/4/09)

Chapter 3

The Provision of Health Care in the United Kingdom

Changes to the provision and delivery of health care in the United Kingdom, particularly since the early 1980s, have been, and still are, rapid and ongoing. This brief introduction to organisation and policy therefore seeks only to act as a useful starting point for developing a more detailed understanding of how the system works.

Outcomes

On completion of this chapter you should be able to:

- identify the main structure and organisation of health and social care provision in the United Kingdom;

- outline the roles and responsibilities of the main organisations in the National Health Service and the independent sector;

- understand the key aims and strategies of current government policy.

INTRODUCTION

The United Kingdom (UK) can be identified as a welfare state, a concept that refers to the state's provision of public measures and support of those in need across society (**www.lse.ac.uk**). Although the state's role in welfare began in the early years of the twentieth century, it was not until after the Second World War that the foundations of the current welfare state were fully established. Measures that were adopted at that time included policy and legislation to deal with what were known then as the interrelated 'five giants of evil', i.e. want (poverty), ignorance (poor education), squalor (lack of and poor housing and town planning), idleness (unemployment) and disease (ill health). The specific policy utilised to combat disease and ill health was the introduction of a National Health Service (NHS). Today, despite many reorganisations and changes, health care in the United Kingdom is still mainly provided through the NHS, although the independent (or private) sector and the voluntary sector are increasingly becoming important partners in the overall provision.

THE NATIONAL HEALTH SERVICE (NHS)

Most formal care in the United Kingdom is provided by the NHS. It was established in 1948 (as part of a welfare state) as a free, comprehensive and universally coordinated health care service, available to the population as a whole. The original structure and organisation lasted until 1974, when the first major changes were made. Since then, in an effort to improve the quality and effectiveness of service provision, considerable and frequent change has taken place. In particular, the service has moved from being centrally directed and organised towards local decision-making, providing a more client-focused service while creating, in theory, greater patient choice.

Today the NHS is a large, complex organisation covering many different services, each of which has different characteristics, different categories of staff and is provided through a variety of organisations. Advances in technology, a growing elderly population, increased expectations and knowledge of service users have all increased the demands for health care, which have to be met out of a limited budget.

The service is still paid for mainly out of general taxation and, with the exception of some dental and optical care and prescribed drugs, it remains free at the point of delivery.

THE NHS ORGANISATION AND STRUCTURE

Prior to 1998 the NHS was organised and managed in the same way across England, Wales, Scotland and Northern Ireland. However, following devolution, there has been an increasing divergence in both policy and structure within each of the countries. Although each of these will be reviewed individually, the main focus for this chapter will be on organisation and management for England.

ENGLAND

Activity

Take a few minutes to consider Figure 1, a diagram of the structure and organisation of the NHS in England.

Figure 1 explained

Department of Health

The Department of Health supports the government to improve the health and well-being of the population. The department provides strategic leadership to the NHS and social care organisations, including:

- setting the overall direction;
- ensuring national standards are met;
- securing resources;
- making major investment decisions;
- improving choice for patients and users;
- improving standards of public health.

Strategic health authorities

The strategic health authorities manage the NHS locally and are the key link between the Department of Health and the NHS. They are charged with:

- ensuring national priorities are integrated into plans for the local health service;
- increasing the capacity of local health services to enable more services to be provided;
- monitoring quality and performance of local health services and developing plans for improvement of health services in their local area.

Primary Care

The term 'primary care' relates to community-based health services that are usually the first and, for some, the only point of contact that patients may have with the health service. It covers services provided by

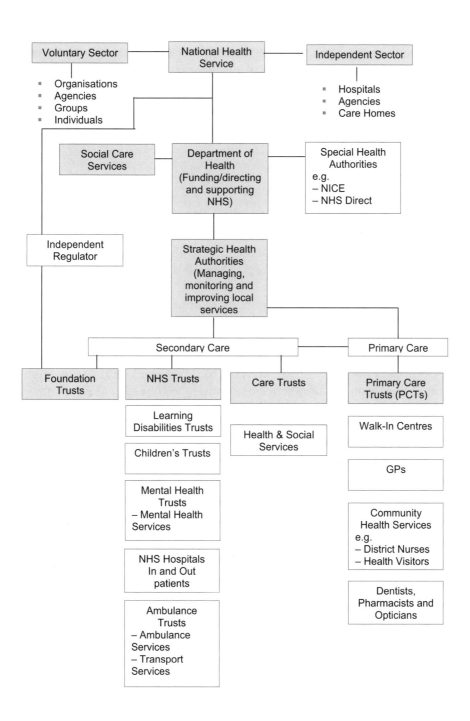

Figure 1 An overview of health care provision (England)

general practitioners (GPs), specialist community public health, family health and general practice nurses, midwives, community therapists (e.g. physiotherapists, occupational therapists), community pharmacists, dentists and optometrists. NHS walk-in centres and NHS Direct are also considered as part of primary care. While primary care is mostly concerned with patients' general health needs, increasingly more specialist treatments and services are becoming available in primary care settings closer to where people live.

Primary Care Trusts

Primary Care Trusts (PCTs) might now be considered the cornerstone of the NHS as they are viewed as the lead in the local health care system and, in England, receive approximately 75–80 per cent of the NHS budget (**www.nhs.uk**). They currently have three main functions.

1. Engaging with their local population to improve health and well-being (in partnership with their local authority). This includes assessing the health needs of all the people in their local area and directly listening to patients' views on services.
2. Commissioning a comprehensive and equitable range of high-quality responsive and efficient services, within allocated resources (these may include services from NHS Trusts, Foundation Trusts, independent hospitals or voluntary services and be from within the United Kingdom or from wider Europe).
3. Monitoring the quality and effectiveness of the services they provide.

Primary Care Trusts are accountable directly to their local population and to their strategic health authority.

NHS Walk-in centres

Walk-in centres give fast access to health advice and treatment for minor illnesses and injuries. The centres are mostly nurse-led units and no appointment is necessary to access the service. Most are open seven days a week from early to late, although a few provide a 24-hour service. They offer a variety of services, which may include:

- assessment by an experienced NHS nurse;
- treatment for minor illnesses and for minor injuries;
- advice on health promotion;
- information on out-of-hours GP and dental services;
- information on local pharmacy services;
- information on other health services.

Where a walk-in centre has been developed by a private company, they remain subject to the same quality monitoring as the NHS.

Secondary care

The term 'secondary care' relates generally to acute hospital and specialist services, the funding of which now comes mainly from the PCTs for commissioned services.

NHS Trusts

NHS Trusts employ the majority of the health service workforce in the UK. Trusts are largely self-governing but are accountable to the strategic health authority for their performance management, and to PCTs for the quality of commissioned health service provision and delivery. Some acute trusts are also regional or national centres for more specialised care, like, for example, renal care.

Foundation Trusts

Foundation Trusts are organisations within the NHS with greater freedom to develop and improve services at a local level and in response to local need. They are seen by the government as being at the forefront of their commitment to the decentralisation of public services and the creation of a patient-led NHS. They are organised as separate entities and are deemed 'public benefit corporations', i.e. they are non-profit-making organisations and are perceived to be owned by their members who are local people, employees and key stakeholders.

Foundation Trusts are not governed by the Department of Health (thereby in theory allowing more freedom) but are accountable to, and must adhere to arrangements made by, an independent regulator who is accountable to Parliament. However, Foundation Trusts are still firmly part of the NHS and are thus still subject to NHS standards, performance ratings and systems of inspection through the Care Quality Commission and through service-level agreements with PCTs and other NHS Trusts.

Care Trusts

Care Trusts were introduced in an attempt to enable closer integration between the health and social care sectors. They may carry out a range of services including social care, mental health services or primary care services. They can be established when NHS organisations and local authorities agree to work in partnership to deliver services. To date relatively few Care Trusts have been established.

Special Health Authorities

These have been established to provide a 'national service' (not just for the local community) to the NHS. They are independent but can be subject to ministerial direction like any other NHS body. They include, for example, the National Institute for Health and Clinical Excellence (NICE) and NHS Direct (**www.nhs.uk**; **www.dh.gov.uk**; RCPG, 2004; Galloway, 2008).

National Institute for Health and Clinical Excellence (NICE)

Established in 2004, NICE was set up as an independent organisation whose overall remit is to bring together knowledge and guidance on ways of promoting good health and treating ill health. Guidance is developed using the expertise of the NHS and wider health care community including NHS staff, health care professionals, patients and carers, industry and the academic world. NICE produces guidance in three areas of health:

1. **Health technologies** – guidance on the use of new and existing medicines, treatments and procedures within the NHS.
2. **Clinical practice** – guidance on the appropriate treatment and care of people with specific diseases and conditions within the NHS.
3. **Public health** – guidance on the promotion of good health and the prevention of ill health for those working in the NHS, local authorities and the wider public and voluntary sector.

www.nice.org.uk

NHS Direct

NHS Direct is perceived by the government as playing a key role in the delivery of 24-hour health advice and information on a range of subjects (for example, self-care, access to local services) to patients and the public. The service provides:

- an established telephone service (0845 4647);
- an online website (**www.nhsdirect.nhs.uk**);
- NHS Direct Interactive – an interactive public service on digital TV – Sky Interactive and Freeview channel 100;
- commissioned services to other parts of the NHS to help meet their patients' needs – these services include:
  - out-of-hours support for GPs and dental services;
  - telephone support for patients with long-term conditions;
  - pre- and post-operative support for patients;
  - 24-hour response to health scares;
  - remote clinics via telephone.

Development of clinical services

Over the last 25 years, successive governments have produced a plethora of policy documents relating to the development of clinical services within the NHS. One such document that is of significant importance and therefore will briefly be considered here is *The NHS Plan: A plan for investment, a plan for reform* (Department of Health, 2000) published in July 2000.

The NHS Plan: A plan for investment, a plan for reform (2000)

Described by the government as the biggest change in health care since the NHS was formed in 1948, this 10-year plan outlined a range of targets and initiatives, some of which were new and some of which reflected earlier commitments. The overall emphasis of the plan was on investment and reform. The key aspects of the plan were that:

- it identified that there would be no changes to the way the NHS was funded but funding would be increased;
- it proposed increases in hospitals, bed capacity, equipment, consultants, GPs, nurses and other health care professionals;
- it gave a commitment to reducing the major causes of mortality and morbidity through the reduction of health inequalities;
- it proposed improving patient access to primary care, and reducing out patient/in patient and accident and emergency waiting times;
- it proposed an expansion of intermediate care facilities, diagnostic and treatment centres, day surgery and short stay treatment;
- it proposed improving joint working between the NHS and other care providers and identified the need to develop a greater role for the private (independent) sector;
- it identified a new performance management system in which Trusts that were judged to have performed well could earn more autonomy on finances and service improvement;
- it proposed the setting of new national standards and a framework to support the delivery of those standards;
- it identified changes to the professions and included new contracts for consultants and GPs, a commitment to give nurses new roles and responsibilities, and improvements in professional regulation;
- it gave a commitment to improve collaboration and teamwork between different professions;
- it put forward plans to improve patient and public involvement at all levels of service provision;
- it gave commitments to improving public health.

(Department of Health, 2000)

A number of these targets and initiatives have already been put into place by the government and you will recognise these within your practice as a student nurse.

Activity

Several other policy documents have also been published linked to *The NHS Plan*. These include:

- *The Health and Social Care (Community Health Standards) Bill* (2003)
- *The NHS Improvement Plan: Putting people at the heart of public services* (2004)
- *Making Partnerships Work for Patients, Carers and Service Users* (2004)
- *Creating a Patient-led NHS* (2005)
- *Health Reform in England: Update and commissioning framework.* (2006)
- *Our Health, Our Care, Our Say: A new direction for community services* (2006)
- Health and Social Care Act (2008)
- *High Quality for All: NHS Next Stage Review Final Report* (2008)

Executive summaries for all of the above can be accessed at **www.dh.gov.uk** and a review of these will provide you with a greater understanding of the current and future developments related to health care provision.

The NHS Constitution

One further document recently published is the new *NHS Constitution*. Published on 21 January 2009, it was one of a number of recommendations in Lord Darzi's report *High Quality Care for All: NHS Next Stage Review Final Report*, which was published on the 60th anniversary of the NHS and set out a ten-year plan to provide the highest quality of care and service for patients in England. The *NHS Constitution* seeks to bring together, in one place for the first time in the history of the NHS, what staff, patients and public can expect from the NHS.

As well as capturing the purpose, principles and values of the NHS, the *Constitution* identifies a number of rights, pledges and responsibilities for staff and patients alike. Subject to parliamentary approval, all NHS bodies and private and third-sector providers supplying NHS services in England will be required by law to take account of the *Constitution* in their decisions and actions. The government will have a legal duty to renew the *Constitution* every 10 years. No government will be able to change the *Constitution*, without the full involvement of staff, patients and the public (**www.dh.gov.uk**).

Activity

It is recommended that an executive summary of this important document is obtained from **www.dh.gov.uk**. Just type 'NHS Constitution' into the site search facility.

Clinical aspects of care

This area will be considered in more detail as you work through this handbook. However, one long-term government policy strategy launched in 1998 that will be considered here is the National Service Frameworks (NSFs).

National Service Frameworks

These frameworks form one of a range of measures that seek to raise quality and decrease variations in service across the NHS. (Variations in service are often referred to as the 'postcode lottery'.) The government strategy through the NSFs so far published has been to:

- set national standards and define the way in which a service should be provided;
- set clear quality requirements for care, based on the best possible evidence of what treatment and services work most effectively for patients;
- offer strategies and support to help health organisations achieve these standards.

Each NSF is developed with the assistance of an external reference group that involves health care professionals, service users and carers, health service managers, partner agencies and other advocates. National Service Frameworks so far established are:

- Mental Health (1999);
- Paediatric Intensive Care (1999);
- Coronary Heart Disease (2000);
- Cancer (2000);
- Older People (2001);
- Diabetes (2001);
- Renal (2004);
- Children (2004);
- Long-term Conditions (2005);
- Chronic Obstructive Pulmonary Disease (COPD) (2008).

National Service Frameworks are relevant to all providers and all deliverers of health care (particularly nurses) in England. (Wales has embraced broadly similar frameworks while Scotland and Northern Ireland have their own system of clinical guidelines and service standards.)

www.dh.gov.uk

Activity

Given the importance of the NSFs you will find it useful to review any of the frameworks identified above when working in that specific area. Further information on each of them can be accessed from **www.dh.gov.uk**. Just type 'National Service Frameworks' in the search box.

WALES

Figure 2 outlines the structure of the NHS in Wales.

Figure 2 explained

The National Assembly (NAW)

In 2006 the Welsh Assembly gained the ability to make its own legislation on devolved matters including health and social care. These are now a new category of Welsh laws called Assembly Measures.

The Welsh Assembly Government is the executive body of the NAW and includes the Minister for Health and Social Services. All NHS statutory organisations in Wales (including the Trusts and Local Health Boards) are accountable to the minister for their performance and the minister is

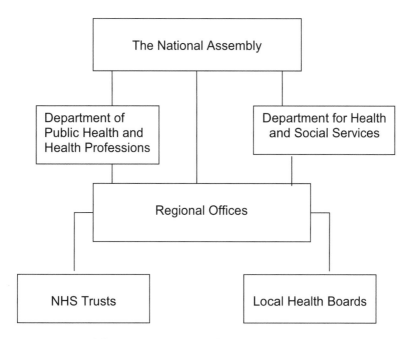

Figure 2 Overview of the current structure of the NHS in Wales

ultimately accountable to the government for the overall running of the Welsh NHS. The Welsh government is responsible for policy direction and dissemination of funds to the health service.

NHS (Wales) Department (NHSD)

The NHSD is an organisational arm of the Welsh Assembly government, responsible for implementing the Assembly's policies and strategies for the management and development of the NHS in Wales. It is led by a director and provides strategic leadership as well as ensuring policy implementation. The department also advises the Minister for Health and Social Services about securing and allocating health resources, while monitoring Local Health Boards and NHS Trust performances.

Department for Public Health and Health Professionals (DPHHP)

The objectives of the DPHHP are to:

- protect the health of the people in Wales and provide preparedness for health emergencies;
- improve the health of people in Wales and reduce inequalities in health;
- provide professional leadership for health and social care.

Department for Health and Social Services (DHSS)

The responsibilities of the DHSS are:

- advising the Welsh Assembly government in setting policies and strategies for health and social care in Wales;
- contributing to making legislation in the field of health and social care;
- providing funding for the NHS and other health and social care bodies;
- managing and supporting the delivery of health and social care services;
- monitoring and promoting improvements in service delivery.

Local Health Boards (LHBs)

Local Health Boards were created to bring greater accountability to the health service in Wales and provide a simplified system for patients to understand while also enabling the service to have a greater representative voice on how it is governed. The LHBs receive a substantial share of the NHS budget for Wales and are therefore the main bodies for commissioning health care. Their responsibilities include:

- commissioning primary, community, and intermediate and secondary care services;
- assessing the health needs of their area and the effectiveness of the local health system.

NHS Trusts

NHS Trusts continue to run hospitals and provide secondary and specialist care. They also provide community services as there are currently no Primary Care Trusts in Wales (**www.wales.gov.uk**; **www.abpi.org.uk**; Galloway, 2008).

Proposed changes to the structure of the NHS in Wales

On 2 April 2008 the Welsh Assembly Government published the *NHS Consultation Paper: Proposals to change the structure of the NHS in Wales*. Following extensive consultation the proposals for the new NHS in Wales were published in November 2008. These proposals include:

- the abolition of all the existing LHBs (currently 22) and the creation of seven new LHBs;

- the abolition of all but two of the existing NHS Trusts (currently 10) with transfer of all the staff and property to the new LHBs, which will have responsibility for the areas in which those Trusts are currently located.

Local Health Boards will become responsible for planning, designing, developing and securing the delivery of primary, community, in-hospital care services and, where appropriate, specialised services for their local population. If accepted by the Welsh Assembly, the proposed start for these changes is October 2009 (**www.wales.nhs.uk**).

Further information

Further and most current information regarding the structure and work of the NHS in Wales can be obtained from **www.wales.nhs.uk** and **www.new.wales.gov.uk**.

Policy

In 2001 *Improving Health in Wales* (the Welsh equivalent of *The NHS Plan* in England) was launched. The document details a ten-year initiative to develop and improve health services in Wales. This includes the development and implementation of the National Service Frameworks. *Design for Life: Creating world class health and social care for Wales in the 21st century* (2005) builds on the policy direction set in 2001 in order to further improve both health and social care in Wales. Both documents are available from **www.wales.nhs.uk**. Wales also embraces guidance from NICE.

SCOTLAND

Figure 3 provides an overview of the NHS in Scotland.

Figure 3 explained

Scottish Parliament

The Scottish Parliament has full legislative power for health in Scotland. This includes overall responsibility for the NHS in Scotland, and public and mental health; the education and training of health professionals; and the terms and conditions of service of NHS staff and general practitioners.

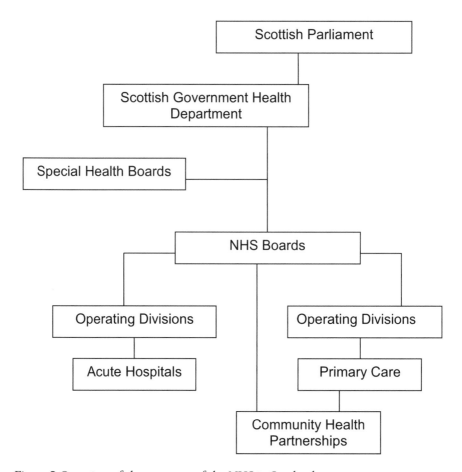

Figure 3 Overview of the structure of the NHS in Scotland

The Scottish Health and Community Department (SHCD)

This department is responsible for determining national objectives and policies for health protection, health improvement and health services, setting targets and offering guarantees on behalf of patients. It is also responsible for providing a statutory and financial framework for NHS Scotland and monitoring quality and value for money.

Special Health Boards

The Special Health Boards provide services across the country and include NHS 24, NHS Quality Improvement Scotland and the Scottish Ambulance Service.

NHS Boards

NHS Boards are responsible for managing local health care organisations and services, allocating funds, monitoring quality, and developing local health care plans in association with local hospitals, GPs and other NHS bodies.

Operating Divisions

Following the abolition of NHS Trusts and Primary Care Trusts in Scotland in 2004, operational management was transferred to operating divisions within the NHS Boards. There are a number of divisions in each board which allocate financial and decision-making powers to the appropriate organisations within their local health care system.

Operating Divisions for Primary Care within the Boards have taken over the responsibilities of the Primary Care Trusts. Their work includes: supporting general practice in the delivery of its services, providing strategic direction and steer service improvement, and work in partnership with local organisations to develop health improvement plans. They are also responsible for monitoring and improving quality and standards in general clinical practice.

Operating Divisions for Secondary Care have operational management responsibilities for the running of hospital services. These functions are devolved under standing orders from the NHS Board.

Community Health Partnerships (CHPs)

Community Health Partnerships are joint organisations comprising local authorities, groups of GPs and other health professionals, in a defined geographic area. The aim of these partnerships is to integrate health services at a local level. Each partnership has a budget for service development to manage their local priorities as described in the local health plan (RCGP, 2004; Galloway, 2008; www.scotland.gov.uk).

Further information

Further current information regarding the structure and work of the NHS in Scotland can be accessed at www.scottish.parliament.uk, www.scotland.gov.uk and www.sehd.scot.nhs.uk

---

Policy in Scotland

In 2000 *Our National Health* (the Scottish equivalent to *The NHS Plan* in England) was launched and in 2007 the *Better Health, Better Care: Action Plan* was published. This document sets out the government's programme to deliver a healthier Scotland by helping people to sustain and improve their health, especially in disadvantaged communities, ensuring better, local and faster access to health care. A copy of both documents is available from **www.scotland.gov.uk**

The National Institute for Health and Clinical Excellence (NICE) does not have a remit in Scotland. Instead, in 2003, NHS Quality Improvement in Scotland was created to provide advice on effective practice; drive and support implementation of improvements in quality; and assess the performance of NHS Scotland reporting and publishing its findings (**www.nhshealthquality.org**).

NHS 24 provides a similar service in Scotland to that of NHS Direct and can be accessed on 08454 242424 or at **www.nhs24.com**

NORTHERN IRELAND

Figure 4 provides an overview of the NHS in Northern Ireland.

Figure 4 explained

Northern Ireland Assembly

The Northern Ireland Assembly has full legislative authority for all 'transferred matters', which include health and social care.

Department of Health, Social Services and Public Safety (DHSSPS)

The DHSSPS is responsible for creating policy and legislation for primary, secondary, community and social care, and for protecting and promoting public health and safety.

The Regional Health and Social Care Board (RHSCB)

The main functions of this board are commissioning, resource management, performance management and improvement of health and social care.

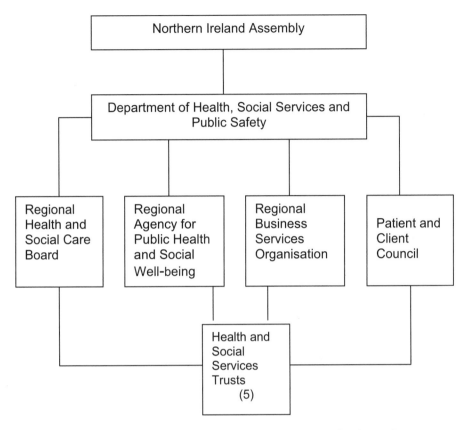

Figure 4 Overview of the structure of the NHS in Northern Ireland (April 2009)

The Regional Agency for Public Health and Social Well-being (RAPHSW)

The broad functions of this agency include responsibility for health protection, health improvement and development to address existing health inequalities and public health issues for the population.

The Regional Business Services Organisation (RBSO)

Set up to provide a range of support functions for health and social care services that include: administrative support; advice and assistance; financial services; human resources; personal and corporate services.

The Patient and Client Council (PCC)

The functions of this council include: representing the interests of the public; promoting the involvement of the public; providing assistance to individuals making or intending to make a complaint relating to health and social care.

Health and Social Services Trusts (HSS Trusts)

Currently there are five HSS Trusts in Northern Ireland. They are charged with delivering a high-quality, cost-effective health and social care service and improving the health and well-being of the population within a given area (**www.northernireland.gov.uk**).

Further information

Further information on the structure and the way in which the NHS works in Northern Ireland can be obtained from **www.healthandcareni.co.uk** or **www.northernireland.gov.uk**

Policy in Northern Ireland

Investing in Health (2002) sets out a plan to improve the health and well-being of the Northern Ireland population (available at **www.investingforhealthni.gov.uk**).

Caring for People Beyond Tomorrow (2005) provides a strategic framework for the development of primary health and social care for individuals, families and communities in Northern Ireland (available from **www.dhssni.gov.uk**).

Health and Social Care (Reform) Act (2009) sets out the legislative framework for structural reform of health and social care in Northern Ireland (available from **www.northernireland.gov.uk**).

Northern Ireland follows NICE guidelines about medication and health procedures and NHS Direct is the same as for England.

(It should be noted that unlike England, Wales, and Scotland, the Northern Ireland health and social services have been integrated as one system since 1972.)

THE INDEPENDENT SECTOR (PRIVATE SECTOR)

According to Baggot (2004), it is difficult to fully estimate the size of the independent sector within the UK due mainly to its diversity.

It consists of large and small private organisations as well as individual practitioners working partly or wholly in a private capacity. It also includes a considerable range of health care services from acute hospitals and care homes through to dentistry and alternative medicine. What further complicates the issue is that patients may also pay privately for some NHS services (for example, treatment in an NHS hospital). Interestingly the NHS is itself one of the largest providers of private medical care with, currently, more NHS Trust private units than any of the private hospital groups (**www.consumerrightsexpert.co.uk**).

While the health care system is still predominantly a public service model it is clear that, overall, the independent sector has become increasingly important over the past three decades in the provision and delivery of health care services. It continues to be viewed by the government as an important partner to the NHS in the quest to deliver more convenient care and choice to NHS patients. Baggott (2004, p. 153) identifies that in 2000 the government sought to improve collaboration by formulating an agreement with the sector (Independent Health Care Association and Department of Health, 2000) that was intended as an enabling framework to foster closer involvement of the independent sector in:

• the planning, commissioning or subcontracting of services from it in order to expand the capacity of the health care system;
• closer cooperation in workforce planning;
• the provision of information on adverse clinical effects, clinical performance and treatment of NHS patients.

Since this agreement there has been the development of the Independent Sector Healthcare Programme, the aim of which is to develop treatment centres that deliver high-quality, cost-effective, scheduled diagnostic and/or treatment services. They are largely run by the private companies in the independent sector, but with operations paid for from NHS funds. They are therefore expected to provide treatment to NHS patients in accordance with NHS principles, with treatment free at the point of delivery and available according to clinical need, not ability to pay. Treatment centres are viewed as playing a key part in the delivery of *The NHS Plan* targets (**www.connectingforhealth.nhs.uk**).

Another recent initiative is that of the Independent Information Project. This project aims to ensure high-quality data for all NHS-funded care by including the private sector within its stakeholder and reference groups (**www.ic.nhs.uk**).

Private health insurance

Although successive governments have actively encouraged the take-up of personal private health insurance, the uptake has remained relatively low and stable. According to Ipsos MORI, only 12 per cent of consumers had private insurance in 2007 and it is forecast that the numbers will only grow slightly between 2007 and 2012 (**www.datamonitor.com**).

Further information

Starting points for further information regarding the independent sector can be found at: **www.hd.gov.uk, www.independenthealthcare.org.uk, www.consumerrightsexpert.co.uk** and **www.ic.nhs.uk/is**

VOLUNTARY CARE SECTOR (VCS)

The voluntary care sector (VCS) has a long tradition of providing services directly to the community and specific client groups, particularly those who often fall outside the so-called mainstream health and social care system. As elsewhere, voluntary organisations range from international organisations with professional staff (for example, the Red Cross), national organisations (for example, the Multiple Sclerosis Society) to small local groups that operate on a largely informal basis.

Like the independent sector, there has been a significant move towards including the VCS in the provision and delivery of health care within the UK. In 2004 representatives from the VCS, health and social care and the Department of Health reviewed ways to further promote an increasing role of the voluntary sector through contribution to health service planning and delivery. There followed a jointly developed agreement between the government, the NHS and the VCS that established a framework of partnership working through the introduction of the National Strategic Partnership Forum (NSPF).

The NSPF

The NSPF is a departmental working group of the Department of Health and reports to ministers. Its membership consists of individuals representing organisations from the VCS, NHS and social care, local government and the Department of Health. The primary principle underpinning the purpose and work of the Forum is the commitment to improving the experience of patients, service users and carers by helping the voluntary, community and public services to work more effectively together (Department of Health, 2005).

Activity

Using a general search engine such as Google, or other information services such as the local library, identify further examples of international, national and locally based voluntary care groups that might support the delivery and provision of health care within the UK.

SOCIAL CARE

Social care in the United Kingdom is another of the major public service areas. In England, the responsibility to provide social care services rests principally with Local Authorities (councils). Since the 1980s there have been numerous government initiatives to integrate the provision and delivery of social and health care more closely, including the introduction of Care Trusts. Providers of social care are now expected to work closely with others, including the NHS, voluntary and independent organisations, as well as the education service, the probation service, the police and other agencies which share the responsibility to provide social care and support. Social care services may be offered in a variety of settings including hospitals, health centres, educational settings, community groups, residential homes, advice centres and in people's own homes.

There are a considerable number of social care services available at most councils and these may include:

- adoption;
- AIDS and HIV;
- care homes;
- carers;
- child protection;
- children in care;
- community development;
- day care;

- elderly people;
- families;
- fostering;
- home adaptations;
- home help;
- learning disabilities;
- leaving hospital;
- mental health;
- occupational therapy;
- personal care at home;
- residential care;
- respite care;
- substance misuse;
- voluntary organisations.

Access to services

Access to social services is normally made by contacting the relevant social care service directly. Information and contact details for care services can usually be found either on the provider council's website, from leaflets at council offices or from local libraries. Alternatively, a GP can refer an individual to the services they require. It should, however, be noted that an individual may need to undergo an assessment to access some services to ensure suitability.

Regulation and monitoring

The Care Quality Commission provides independent monitoring regarding both quality and performance of the whole health and adult social care sector (a brief overview of the commission's work can be found in Chapter 7 on 'Quality assurance').

Future plans

The government is to publish a Green Paper on the future shape of the social care and support system in 2009.

Further information

Further information regarding the provision of social care within the UK can be accessed from **www.dh.gov.uk**, **www.nhs.uk** and **www.dh.gov.uk/en/socialcare/index.htm**. The latter provides an overview of national policy, practical guidance and standards for the social care sector.

REFERENCES

Baggot, R. (2004) *Health and Health Care in Britain* (3rd edn). New York: Palgrave Macmillan

Department of Health (2000) *The NHS Plan: A plan for investment; a plan for reform*. London: Department of Health

Department of Health (2005) *National Strategic Partnership Forum – Statement of Purpose*. London: Department of Health

Department of Health (2006) *Health Reform in England: Update and commissioning framework*. London: Department of Health.

Galloway, M. (2008) *The ACP Guide to the Structure of the NHS in the United Kingdom*. East Sussex: Association of Clinical Pathologists

Royal College of General Practitioners (2004) *The Structure of the NHS: Information Sheet No. 8*. London: RCGP

Scottish Executive (2000) *Our National Health: A plan for action, a plan for change*. Edinburgh: Scottish Executive

Welsh Assembly Government (2001) *Improving Health in Wales*. Cardiff: National Assembly

Useful websites

www.nice.org.uk (accessed 2/2/09)

www.lse.ac.uk/resources/LSEHistory/beveridge_report.htm (accessed 2/2/09)

www.dh.gov.uk/en/Healthcare/NHSConstitution/index.htm (accessed 1/2/09)

www.nhs.uk (accessed 31/1/09)

www.dh.gov.uk (accessed 31/1/09)

www.wales.gov.uk/about/departments/dhss/?lang=en (accessed 30/1/09)

www.abpi.org.uk/wales_nhs.asp (accessed 1/2/09)

www.wales.nhs.uk/sites3/page.cfmorgid=222&pid=31302 (accessed 29/1/09)

www.scottish.parliament.uk/business/research/pdf_subj_maps/
   smda-08.pdf (accessed 20/1/09)
www.scotland.gov.uk (accessed 29/1/09)
www.sehd.scot.nhs (accessed 1/2/09)
www.northernireland.gov.uk (accessed 1/2/09)
www.healthandcareni.co.uk (accessed 1/2/09)
www.nhshealthquality.org/nhsqis (accessed 29/1/09)
www.datamonitor.com/Products/Free/Report/
   DMF52168/020DMF2168 (accessed 2/2/09)
www.consumerrightsexpert.co.uk/PrivateHealthCare (accessed 2/2/09)
www.ic.nhs.uk/is (accessed 2/2/09)
www.connectingforhealth.nhs.uk/systemsandservices/ishealthcarepro
   (accessed 2/2/09)

Chapter 4

Legal and Professional Issues

The aim of this chapter is to make you aware of the legal and professional issues surrounding nursing. You may not feel that all the considerations below apply to you as you are not an NMC registrant (yet). However, as a citizen or resident of the UK the legal aspects do apply (criminal and civil law). In addition you are advised to look on the NMC regulations as a guide to best practice. Any employment regulation may affect you when undertaking clinical practice and you should also be aware of any charters, guidelines, policies etc., that your university, college and/or placement organisation asks you to respect.

Outcomes

On completion of this chapter you should be able to:

- demonstrate an awareness of the legal framework within which care is provided;

- discuss the legal responsibilities of nurses when caring for patients or clients;

- define the term 'accountability' in relation to *The Code: Standards of conduct, performance and ethics* (NMC, 2008a) and other guidelines issued by the NMC.

ACCOUNTABILITY

'To be accountable is literally to be liable to be called upon to give an account of what one has done or not done' (Banks, 2004, p. 150). The importance of accountability in professional life is not new, but there is an increasing focus on issues surrounding nursing accountability and nurses, both registered and in training, must be aware of the implications it brings.

Accountability is often defined as responsibility, but there is a difference between the two. Responsibility is concerned with answering for what you do, whereas accountability is being answerable for the 'consequences' of what you do. The most important factor in accountability is that it is 'personal' and no registered nurse can be accountable for another. The NMC (2008a, p.1) states this very clearly in *The Code: Standards of conduct, performance and ethics* (hereafter referred to as *The Code*):

> As a professional, you are personally accountable for actions and omissions in your practice and must always be able to justify your actions.

> You must always act lawfully, whether those laws relate to your professional practice or personal life.

As a student nurse you are not 'professionally accountable' in the way that you will be after registering with the NMC (NMC, 2005). This means you cannot be called upon to account for your actions and omissions with the NMC. As far as the NMC is concerned, it is the registered nurses with whom you work who are professionally responsible for the consequences of your actions and omissions. This is why you must always work under direct supervision.

Activity

Visit the NMC website (**www.nmc-uk.org**) and download and read: *An NMC guide for students of nursing and midwifery* (2005). This sets out your responsibilities as a student.

Castledine (1991) offers a further definition of accountability that, although written some time ago, is still very pertinent today as it encompasses the whole ethos of how accountability in nursing should be viewed. He states accountability is:

> that phenomena related to nursing practice which nurses are entrusted with, are answerable for, take the credit and the blame for, and can be judged within legal and moral boundaries.
>
> Castledine (1991, p. 28)

It is these legal boundaries that this chapter explores.

Arenas of accountability

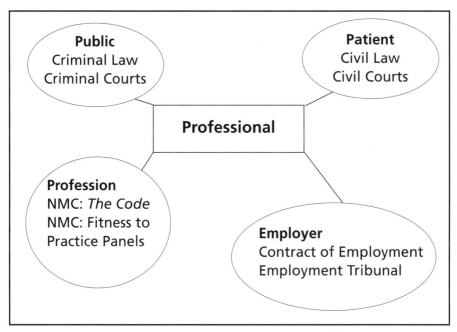

Figure 1 Arenas of accountability (adapted from Dimond, 2005)

As you can see from Figure 1, Dimond (2005), a barrister who has a great interest in professional accountability and patients' rights, believes there are four arenas of accountability that nurses must consider. Certainly the public, patient and employment sections apply to you as a student nurse.

Criminal law and the courts

In criminal law a crime is committed against the state, either when an act is performed that the law forbids, or when an act is omitted that the law requires. For a conviction it must be proved that a person intended to commit the crime, or was reckless in doing the criminal act. More serious cases include murder, manslaughter and rape (all of which nurses have been found guilty of) and are heard in crown courts before a judge and jury. Lesser cases (for example driving offences) are heard in a magistrates' court. The outcome of prosecution is a custodial sentence or fine.

Civil law and the courts

This part of the law involves the rights and duties individuals have towards each other. Legal action can be taken by a private individual against another individual or an organisation. This is the main legal area that affects nurses and which lawyers refer to as the law of torts. The outcomes from these cases usually involve awards of compensation (for damages) or orders (injunctions) to stop an individual acting unlawfully. It is interesting to note that the NMC recognises that this is an area where nurses are increasingly being involved and, from 2004, it has included a section in *The Code* in which it recommends registered nurses have professional indemnity insurance – 'in the event of claims of professional negligence' (NMC, 2008a, p. 11).

Duty of care (negligence)

An action for negligence is a civil action, and results from a breach of duty of care. A nurse may be held legally liable if it can be shown that either they have failed to exercise the skills properly expected of them, or that they have undertaken tasks that they are not competent to perform (Dimond, 2005). For negligence to be proved three conditions must be satisfied:

1. a duty of care is owed by the defendant (nurse) to the plaintiff (patient), i.e. the nurse/patient relationship;
2. there is a breach in the standard of care;
3. this breach has caused harm either by action or omission.

Some criminal cases may also have a civil action brought against them if any harm has been caused by 'action or omission'.

Activity

- Think of a circumstance where a nurse might be held criminally liable (i.e. a criminal act that a nurse might commit).
- Think of circumstances in clinical practice where a nurse may be judged negligent (i.e. perform an act that could be referred to a civil court).

Accountability to the employer

All those in a nursing role are accountable to their employer. There is an implied term in every contract of employment that the employee will obey the reasonable instructions of the employer (i.e. follow any policies, procedures, standards, etc.), and that any employee who breaches their contract may be subject to disciplinary action. Even though, as a student nurse, you are not 'employed' by a placement organisation as such, you are still bound by their 'instructions', and any deviation from this could lead to disciplinary action by your university and/or your placement provider. This means you must be familiar with their policies, procedures, etc., and act in accordance with them. The NMC (2005) confirms this when it says that 'you [student nurses] can be called to account by your university or by the law for the consequences of your actions or omissions as a pre-registration student'.

Vicarious liability

An employer is liable for civil actions (torts) committed by their employees (for example, nurses) during the scope of their employment, However, this does not remove any legal responsibility/accountability from the nurse (Dimond, 2005). The employer (for example the NHS Trust/care home) cannot shirk this liability by saying it provides competent, trained staff – it will always be primarily responsible for any negligence to patients by their staff.

However, if a patient takes a civil action against an employer for damages caused by one of its employees, and the employer is found directly liable by the civil courts, the employer could in turn take out an action against the employee. This usually happens when an employer has to pay out compensation to a patient as a result of an employee's negligence, and tries to recoup their money from the employee. As this pertains to civil law, which is applicable to all citizens and residents of the UK, this could affect you as a student nurse.

Professional liability (see also the later section on the NMC)

As a student nurse you are not accountable to the NMC but, as a registered nurse, you will be. Therefore, you must be aware of the professional accountability you will automatically assume when registered. The NMC emphasises the need for all registered nurses and midwives to be personally accountable for their practice by issuing them with *The Code*. Although this document is not part of law (Burnard and Chapman, 2003), the functions of the NMC include a requirement to establish and improve standards of training and professional conduct (Nursing and Midwifery Order, 2001), and they do this by issuing *The Code* and a requirement for all registered nurses to abide by it. Therefore, *The Code* acts as a reminder of the standards required by registered nurses. However, breaching *The Code* is in effect a breach of registration and may lead to the removal of the nurse's name from the register, and consequently the right to practice (Peate, 2006). This is emphasised in *The Code* (NMC, 2008a, p. 1):

Failure to comply with this Code of Conduct may bring your fitness to practice into question and endanger your registration.

Paramount in *The Code*, along with the registered nurse's need to be accountable for their practice, is the mandatory requirement for them to have the knowledge and skills for safe and effective practice (NMC, 2008a, p. 7). In line with this the NMC warns that careful consideration must be made of professional accountability if nurses are asked to work in an area for which they are not adequately prepared – being open about their limitations is not a sign of weakness but rather a key indicator of mature and caring practice (Richards and Edwards, 2008). *The Code* endorses this by stating:

You must recognize and work within the limits of your competence.

You must take part in appropriate learning and practice activities that maintain and develop your competence and performance.

The NMC acknowledges that as a student you will come into close contact with patients, either through observing care being given, through helping provide the care and, towards the end of your course, through full participation in providing care. The NMC states that: 'at all times, you should work only within your level of understanding and competence, and always under the appropriate supervision of a registered nurse' (NMC, 2005, p. 2).

Further to *The Code*, the NMC issues *Standards for medicines management* (NMC, 2007), *Record Keeping Guidance* (2007) and *The Prep (Post-Registration Education and Practice) Handbook* (2008c) to all registered nurses. While, again, these documents have no legal force in themselves, their recommendations are firm guidelines to all nurses who require clear evidence to justify any actions.

Providing care in an emergency situation outside the work environment

The NMC (2008d) recently issued an advice sheet on providing care in an emergency situation outside the workplace. This spans all the areas of accountability registered nurses are concerned with (criminal, civil, employment and professional law), and as students you should be aware of the implications for you.

In the United Kingdom there is generally no legal obligation on a person to provide care or assistance in an emergency situation. However, in an emergency, in or outside the work setting, registered nurses have a professional duty to provide care. The NMC points out (NMC, 2008d) that in providing emergency care, registered nurses are personally accountable for any actions or omissions in their practice, and would be judged against what could reasonably be expected from someone with their knowledge, skills and abilities when placed in those circumstances. The registered nurse would need to ensure that this is within the limits of their competence and that they are able to demonstrate that they acted in the person's best interests (NMC, 2008d).

The NMC (2005) acknowledges that student nurses may be placed in emergency situations on occasion, but advises that 'you do not participate in any procedure for which you have not been fully prepared or in which you are not adequately supervised' (NMC, 2005, p. 3).

Further reading

This section has given a very brief introduction to the law in the United Kingdom. Further detail can be found in a variety of texts written for nurses, perhaps the most comprehensive being those written by Bridgit Dimond (2005), *Legal Aspects of Nursing*, and Helen Caulfield (2005), *Accountability*.

THE NURSING AND MIDWIFERY COUNCIL

The core function of the NMC is to establish standards of education, training, conduct and performance for nursing and midwifery and to ensure those standards are maintained, thereby safeguarding the health and well-being of the public. The powers of the NMC are set out in the Nursing and Midwifery Order 2001. As you can see, although still a student nurse, you are already affected by the role of the NMC as it sets the standards of education and training you are undertaking. They determine the level of entry and content of pre-registration nursing programmes, and universities have to have validation from the NMC to run their programmes. Pre-registration programmes are also monitored and reviewed by them on a regular basis. The NMC's key tasks are to:

- maintain a register of nurses and midwives eligible to practise in the UK;

- set standards and information for nursing and midwifery conduct, performance and ethics;
- quality-assure nursing and midwifery education;
- consider allegations of misconduct, lack of competence or unfitness to practise due to ill health;
- set standards and provide guidance for local supervising authorities for midwives.

www.nmc-uk.org

All nurses in the UK working in a registered nurse capacity must be registered with the NMC. When you have successfully completed your nursing programme, your university will notify the NMC that you have met the required standards and that you are eligible for entry on the register. Your course director will also complete a declaration of good health and good character on your behalf, which must be received by the NMC before registration can take place (NMC, 2005, p.1).

What constitutes good health and good character? (NMC, 2008b)

Good health

Good health is necessary to undertake practice as a nurse or midwife. 'Good health' means that you must be capable of safe and effective practice without supervision. It does not mean the absence of any disability or health condition. Many disabled people and those with long-term health conditions are able to practice with or without adjustments to support their practice. Long-term conditions such as epilepsy, diabetes or depression can be well managed and would then not be incompatible with registration. Temporary health conditions do not necessarily mean a person is not fit to practice. For example, having a broken leg may mean a person is not fit to work for a period of time. It does not mean they are not fit to practice as they can reasonably expect to recover fully and return to work.

Good character

Good character is important as nurses and midwives must be honest and trustworthy. Your good character is based on your conduct, behaviour and attitude. It covers examples such as someone who knowingly practices as a nurse or midwife before they are on the register, or someone who signs a student off from an educational programme while being aware of poor behaviour. It also includes any convictions and cautions that are not considered compatible with professional registration and that might bring the profession into disrepute. Your character must be sufficiently good for you to be capable of safe and effective practice without supervision.

Activity

Visit the NMC website (**www.nmc-uk.org**) and look under 'Registration/Join the register/good health and good character' and look at the scenarios posted there.

Once qualified, nurses will be placed on the register, the sections of which are shown in Figure 2 (**www.nmc-uk.org** 2008).

Registerable qualifications – 1st Level Nurses – Sub-part 1
Adult
Mental Health
Learning Disabilities
Children

Specialist community public health nurses
Specialist Community Public Health Nursing – Health Visitor
Specialist Community Public Health Nursing – School Nurse
Specialist Community Public Health Nursing – Occupational Health Nurse
Specialist Community Public Health Nursing – Family Health Nurse

Recorded qualifications
Mode 1 Prescribing
Extended Nurse Prescribing
Extended/Supplementary Nursing Prescribing
Teacher
Specialist Practitioner – Adult Nursing
Specialist Practitioner – Mental Health
Specialist Practitioner – Children's Nursing
Specialist Practitioner – Learning Disability Nurse
Specialist Practitioner – General Practice Nursing
Specialist Practitioner – Community Mental Health Nursing
Specialist Practitioner – Community Learning Disabilities Nursing
Specialist Practitioner – Community Children's Nursing
Specialist Practitioner – District Nursing

Figure 2 The structure of the NMC Register of Qualified Nurses

The Code: Standards of conduct, performance and ethics for nurses and midwives (2008)

As previously stated, the primary role of the NMC is to safeguard the health and well-being of the public. The way the NMC fulfils this function, designated to it under the Health Act 1999 and the Nursing and Midwifery Order 2001, is to issue all registered nurses and midwives with *The Code. The Code* sets out a minimum standard of behaviour expected of all registered nurses and midwives and, if these standards are not met, nurses and midwives may receive an allegation of unfitness to practice. As students you cannot be disciplined by the NMC using *The Code* but, nevertheless, you are advised to view its contents as best practice and should adhere to its principles when on placement.

The Code is divided into four sections with a number of subsections. The whole code is prefixed with the words (NMC, 2008a, p.1):

> The people in your care must be able to trust you with their health and well-being. To justify that trust, you must . . .

And then indicates the four main sections:

- make the care of people your first concern, treating them as individuals and respecting their dignity;
- work with others to protect and promote the health and well-being of those in your care, their families and carers, and the wider community;
- provide a high standard of practice and care at all times;
- be open and honest, act with integrity and uphold the reputation of your profession.

The introduction continues:

> As a professional, you are personally accountable for actions and omissions in your practice and must always be able to justify your decisions.

> You must always act lawfully, whether those laws relate to your professional practice or personal life.

> Failure to comply with this Code of Conduct may bring your fitness to practice into question and endanger your registration.

This code of conduct should be considered together with the NMC's rules, standards, guidance and advice available from **www.nmc-uk.org**.

DELEGATION

Although *The Code* emphasises that all registered nurses are personally accountable for their practice, there may be some instances where nurses may be delegated tasks, or indeed delegate tasks themselves. The NMC has a section in *The Code* (NMC, 2008a, p. 6) outlining the considerations nurses must take before delegating:

- you must establish that anyone you delegate to is able to carry out your instructions;
- you must confirm that the outcome of any delegated task meets the required standards;
- you must make sure that everyone you are responsible for is supervised and supported.

This last clause could affect you if you believe that a registered nurse has delegated you a task and is not supporting or supervising you. As already mentioned, the NMC states (about students) that: 'at all times, you should work only within your level of understanding and competence, and always under the appropriate supervision of a registered nurse' (NMC, 2005, p. 2). However, the NMC (NMC, 2005, p. 3) does acknowledge:

> there may be times when you are in a position where you may not be directly accompanied by your mentor, supervisor or another registered colleague, such as emergency situations. As your skills, experience and confidence develop, you will become increasingly able to deal with these situations. However, as a student, do not participate in any procedure for which you have not been fully prepared or in which you are not adequately supervised. If such a situation arises, discuss the matter as quickly as possible with your mentor or personal tutor.

Peate (2006) reminds registered nurses of the legal perspective on delegation, and believes that when delegating a task the following must be borne in mind:

- when working as a team member you are personally accountable for your own actions or omissions – there is no such concept as team negligence. If harm occurs, you are individually accountable;

- you must make it known and obtain help and supervision from a competent practitioner if you feel an aspect of practice lies beyond your level of competence or outside your area of registration.

As previously identified, *The Code* (NMC, 2008) is divided into sections. The following pages look at some of the issues *The Code* raises in more detail; those of consent, confidentiality, record-keeping and maintaining professional knowledge and competence.

Case study

Obtain a copy of *The Code* from the NMC website (**www.nmc-uk.org**). Read *The Code*, and then read the following article and identify the sections of *The Code* you think Jo breached – the answers are at the end of the text. (Reproduced with permission from *British Journal of Nursing*.)

STAFF NURSE WHO FAILED TO PROVIDE ADEQUATE NURSING CARE FOR PATIENTS

British Journal of Nursing, 2004, 13 (7): 389 Professional Misconduct Series

In the following case a senior nurse called Jo deliberately ignored certain aspects of care while on night duty because she felt that it was not her responsibility to do certain tasks or check that they had been carried out.

Jo worked on nights for a large inner-city hospital trust and had been doing so for over ten years. When working on the general medical/surgical wards she was often heard to say derogatory remarks about some of the patients or core nursing tasks she was expected to do. For example, she saw it as a junior nursing role to go around and attend to patients' pressure needs. She felt her expertise lay in giving out drugs, managing intravenous infusion lines and doing certain nursing procedures.

On the particular ward where she was working, two patients requested pain relief. Jo did not bother to go and see the patients, but instructed two health care assistants who were on duty with her to give each of the patients two paracetamol tablets. The health care assistants gave the medication to the patients as directed, but at no time did Jo attempt to check what they had given or to clarify with the patients how they were feeling. The situation continued for several shifts. Any patient who required additional pain relief was referred by the health care assistants to Jo, who told them to give paracetamol.

On the last occasion that Jo and the health care assistants were on duty together, an agency nurse was also present because of the workload on the ward. However, Jo still did not help unless she felt it was absolutely necessary. At one time during the evening she left the ward for a break, stating that she had left the keys on the shelf in the office. These keys included keys to the controlled drug cupboard and the drugs trolley. Although Jo was entitled to a break from the ward, this was the third she had taken that night and she did not tell the staff where she was going.

The agency nurse was angry that Jo had left the ward without informing her of where she was going and how she could be contacted. Jo also did not tell the agency nurse where she could find the keys. A patient then complained of pain and the health care assistant asked the agency nurse, who was a registered nurse, if she could give the patient some paracetamol. The agency nurse then questioned the health care assistants about the procedure they had been following with Jo.

When Jo eventually returned to the ward, the agency nurse challenged her about the drug administration and leaving the keys in the ward office. Jo was offhand with the agency nurse and did not speak to her for the rest of the shift. At the handover to the day staff, Jo gave the report without involving the rest of the night nursing team. She let the health care assistants and the agency nurse write up the nursing records, but at no time in the handover did she involve them in the verbal report.

The agency nurse complained to the ward manager about the incidents that had occurred, and also some problems relating to a blood transfusion that Jo had been managing. It appeared that Jo had not followed the trust protocol with regard to administration of a transfusion. There had been a long delay before it had been commenced and Jo had not recorded any observations of the patient during the transfusion.

Conclusion

An investigation was carried out by the Trust and it was felt that Jo should be dismissed from her post and her case referred to the NMC. Jo was charged by the NMC and found guilty of:

- failing to provide adequate support for patients on a ward;
- giving medication to health care assistants to administer to patients;
- leaving a ward without advising staff of her whereabouts, and not handing over the ward keys to a registered nurse colleague;
- failing to provide an adequate and appropriate handover of patient care;
- failing to follow the correct protocol and procedure while administering a blood transfusion.

Her name was removed from the nursing register.

Note: this case is in a series based on true cases that were reported to the NMC. Compiled by George Castledine, Professor and Consultant of General Nursing, University of Central England, Birmingham, and Dudley Group of Hospitals NHS Trust.

CONSENT

Every adult, mentally competent person has the right in law to consent to any touching of his/her person, or to refuse any examination or treatment. If he/she is touched without consent or other lawful justification, then the person has the right to bring a criminal action for battery or a civil action for trespass to the person (Dimond, 2005). Furthermore, should harm occur to the patient, it could result in a legal action against the nurse for negligence. Consent also affirms the person's right to self-determination and autonomy (Caulfield, 2005). Lord Donaldson points out that consent is twofold – firstly to obtain 'legal' justification for care (as above), and secondly 'clinical' consent to secure the patient's trust and co-operation.

The NMC (2008a, p. 4) states that as a registered nurse 'you must ensure that you gain consent before any treatment or care'. It also states that it is a professional duty that any information given to allow the patient to make an informed decision must be accurate and truthful and presented in such a way as to make it easily understood.

Consent can be written, verbal or implied ('by co-operation'). They are all equally valid. However, they vary considerably in their value as evidence in proving that consent was given. Consent in writing is the best form of evidence and therefore is the preferred method for patients when any procedure involving some risk is contemplated. As a student you would not be expected to give information to patients regarding their condition or treatment or obtain any written consent, but any form of nursing intervention requires their consent. When referring to students the NMC (2005, p. 2) points out:

> You must respect the wishes of patients and clients at all times.
> They have the right to refuse to allow you, as a student, to
> participate in caring for them and you should make this right
> clear to them when they are first given information about the care
> they will receive from you. You should leave if they ask you to do
> so. Their rights, as patients or clients, supersede at all times your
> rights to knowledge and experience.

It must be remembered that it is a basic principle of law in this country that an adult, mentally competent person has the right to refuse treatment and take his or her own discharge contrary to medical advice. The NMC (2008a, p. 4) supports this when stating 'you must respect and support people's rights to accept or decline treatment and care'. Consent must be:

- given by a legally competent person;
- informed;
- given freely.

A legally competent person

The person giving consent must have the capacity to do so. A legally competent person must be able to understand and retain information and use the information to make an informed decision. You must presume that a patient is competent unless otherwise assessed by a suitably qualified practitioner. The assessment as to whether an adult lacks the capacity to consent is made by the clinician providing treatment or care, but should also involve nurses' views.

No one has the right to consent on behalf of another competent adult. Further, it is accepted that adults over the age of 16 have the relevant capacity to understand and make their own decisions about medical and nursing treatment (Caufield, 2005).

Adults temporarily unable to consent

In emergency situations where an adult becomes unable to consent (for example, due to being unconscious), the law allows treatment as long as it is 'in the patient's best interests'. Medical intervention that can be delayed until the patient can consent should be delayed (exceptions to this are when the person has issued an advanced directive refusing treatment). In 'the patient's best interests' is said to be when a 'body of other similar treatment providers would also give the same treatment' (Tingle and Cribb, 2006, p. 168), and arises from a court case in 1989 (*F* v. *West Berkshire Health Authority*).

Informed consent

The patient must be able to give informed consent to the proposed treatments and the information, given by any health care professional (including registered nurses) should include any material risks like, for example, the nature and consequences of the proposed treatment, and the consequences of not having the treatment and any alternatives to the treatment.

Given freely

Consent must be given freely – this means that no threats or implied threats must be used, that no 'coercion and undue influence' is applied. Coercion invalidates consent, and if a nurse feels that the patient is being coerced, either by another health care professional or family member, they should seek to see the patient alone to ascertain that their wishes are being adhered to (Peate, 2006).

Children and young people

If the patient is under 18 years old (age of consent) the rules concerning consent are different. A person aged 16–17 is allowed to consent to treatment under the Family Law Reform Act (1979), in a similar way to an adult. However, refusal of treatment can be overridden by a person with parental authority or a court order.

A person under the age of 16 years, who has sufficient understanding and intelligence to enable them to understand the proposed treatment or investigation, may have the capacity to consent (Department of Health, 2001). Children who have these capacities are said to be 'Gillick competent' (Peate, 2006). The term Gillick (sometimes referred to as 'Fraser' after the judge who heard the case) comes from a court case in 1985 that concerned a teenage girl's right to consent to medical treatment without her parents' knowledge (*Gillick* v. *West Norfolk and Wisbech Area Health Authority*). An assessment to determine whether a minor is Gillick (Fraser) competent must ask the following questions (Peate, 2006, p. 72).

- Does the child understand the proposed treatment, his/her medical condition, and the consequences that may emerge if he/she refuses or agrees to treatment?
- Does he/she understand the moral, social and family issues involved in the decision he/she is to make?
- Does the mental state of the child fluctuate?
- What treatment is to be performed – does the child understand the complexities of the proposed treatment and the potential risks associated with it?

Mental Capacity Act (2005)

The Mental Capacity Act became law in 2007 and affects people living in England and Wales over the age of 16. It is concerned with protecting the public who lack capacity to make their own decisions about a variety of health and social circumstances. The Act introduces:

- a new test to determine 'a person's best interests';
- new Lasting Powers Of Attorney that extend to a person's health and welfare as well as property and money;
- a new Court of Protection and a new office of Public Guardian to support the Court;
- deputies who can make decisions in the 'person's best interests';
- a new criminal offence of ill-treatment and neglect;
- regulation of advance decisions to refuse treatment;
- regulation of research in relation to individuals who lack mental capacity;
- a new Independent Mental Capacity Advocate service (IMCA) for people with no family or friends;
- a Code of Practice to accompany the Act – health care professionals will have a duty to abide by the Code.

Underlying principles of the Mental Capacity Act (2005) (www.ncpc.org.uk)

- A presumption of capacity: everyone has the right to their own decisions, so a person must be assumed to have capacity unless it is established that they lack capacity.
- Individuals should be supported where possible so that they can make their own decisions: a person must not be treated as being unable to make a decision unless all practicable steps to help them to do so have been taken, without success.
- People have the right to make decisions that may seem eccentric or unwise to other people: a person is not to be treated as unable to make a clear decision merely because he or she makes an unwise decision.
- Best interests: acts done or decisions made on behalf of a person established to be lacking capacity must be in their best interests.
- Rights and freedoms must be restricted as little as possible: before doing an act or taking a decision on behalf of a person, regard must be had as to whether the purpose underlying that act or decision can be achieved in a way less restrictive of his rights or freedom of action.

A person who lacks capacity:

- is unable to make a decision for themselves by reason of disturbance of their mind or brain, whether on a temporary or permanent basis;
- is unable to make a decision if they cannot understand relevant information, retain that information, use or weigh that information as part of making a decision, or is unable to communicate their decision 'by any means'.

Lack of capacity cannot be established merely by reference to a person's age, appearance, or behaviour.

Advance decisions to refuse treatment

The Mental Capacity Act 2005 allows patients over the age of 18 years to state, in writing, in advance what treatment they would not like carried out should they become unable to decide for themselves. These decisions must be respected by all health care professionals, which obviously includes nurses. The person must be deemed competent when making the advance directive, and only clear refusals of specific treatments will be upheld (surgery, drug therapy, etc.). If any doubt exists, then treatment may be given 'in the patient's best interests'. Furthermore, a patient cannot refuse basic care.

Mental Health Acts

For people detained under relevant mental health legislation, the principles of consent continue to apply for all conditions not related to the mental disorder.

Further information

Further information about consent can be obtained from the Department of Health website at **www.dh.gov.uk** (type 'consent' in the main search engine). Key guidance includes:

- a reference guide to the principles on consent to examination and treatment;
- good practice in consent implementation guide.

In addition, on the same website, there is information about consent forms and associated guidance for patients. Another website pertaining to the Mental Capacity Act (2005) is **www.dca.gov.uk** (type 'mca' into search engine).

CONFIDENTIALITY

Confidentiality is a fundamental part of the patient/client relationship. Any information given to a nurse by a patient should not be passed on to anyone outside the health care team without consent. The fundamental importance of trust between a health professional and the patient brings with it a 'duty of confidence' (Caulfield, 2005). This duty arises from:

- duty of care in negligence (discussed earlier in the chapter) – a breach of confidentiality can lead to civil action;
- implied duties under the nurse's contract of employment;
- requirements of the NMC outlined in *The Code* – a breach of this could result in removal from the nurses' register.

The NMC endorses Caulfield's statements in its section of *The Code* by stating (NMC, 2008a, p. 2):

- you must respect people's right to confidentiality;
- you must ensure people are informed about how and why information is shared by those who will be providing care.

Furthermore *The Code* states:

- you must disclose information if you believe someone may be at risk of harm, in line with the law of the country in which you are practising.

Disclosing information

NMC guidance (NMC, 2007) clearly states that disclosure of confidential information without consent should only happen in exceptional circumstances. Nurses must be able to justify their actions in doing so, and it must only be done in the public interest to protect individuals, groups or society as a whole from the risk of significant harm. Examples could include child abuse, serious crime or drug trafficking. If a decision to disclose is made, a clear and accurate account should be recorded in the person's records.

Dimond (2005) summarises this when stating there are seven exceptions to the duty of confidence, when nurses can divulge information about their patients:

- with the patient's consent;
- in the patient's best interests;
- by court order;
- under statutory duty to disclose;
- in the public's interests;
- to the police;
- under provisions within the Data Protection Act 1998.

Confidentiality does not only apply within a health care setting. As a student you may wish to refer to a real-life situation that you have been involved with in an academic assignment. If so, your university will have guidelines on confidentiality, which you must abide by and which will advise you not to provide any information that could identify a particular patient.

Ownership of and access to records (NMC, 2007)

Records of information belong to an organisation (for example a hospital) and not to specific people. People can, however, request to see their paper-held and computer-held notes. The Data Protection Act 1998, the Access Modification Health Order 1987, Access to Medical Reports

Act 1990, and the Access to Health Records (Northern Ireland) Order 1993 define their rights to access. Procedures for access must be made in accordance with the Freedom of Information Act 2000 and the Freedom of Information (Scotland) Act 2002.

- The Data Protection Act 1998 gives the patient a statutory right to access personal information in the form of health records held on them (both computer and manually-held records). The definition of 'health record' includes all records relating to their health, for example nursing records, physiotherapy records, laboratory results, etc. The patient also has the right of rectification (make right/amend) if the data recorded appear to be inaccurate.
- The Access to Medical Reports Act 1988 gives an individual the right of access to any medical report relating to them supplied for employment purposes or insurance purposes.
- The Access to Health Records Act 1990 governs access to health records of deceased people.
- The Freedom of Information Act 2000 and Freedom of Information Act (Scotland) 2002 grant anyone the right to information that is not covered by the Data Protection Act 2000 (i.e. information that does not contain a person's identifiable details).

Caldicott

A review was commissioned in 1997 by the Chief Medical Officer of England due to:

> increasing concern about the ways in which patient information is being used in the NHS in England and Wales and the need to ensure that confidentiality is not undermined. Such concern was largely due to the development of information technology in the service, and its capacity to disseminate information about patients rapidly and extensively.
>
> (Department of Health, 1999)

As a result of the report every NHS organisation is required to appoint a 'Caldicott Guardian' who is responsible for agreeing and reviewing internal protocols governing the protection and use of patient-identifiable information by the staff of their organisations.

Further information

Further information about confidentiality can be obtained from the Department of Health website at **www.dh.gov.uk** (type 'confidentiality NHS code of practice' in the main search engine). Key guidance includes:

- what is confidential information?;
- providing a confidential service;
- legal requirements;
- a list of confidentiality decisions.

RECORD-KEEPING

Record-keeping is part of the professional duty of care owed by the registered nurse to the patient. As a student you can take part in record-keeping activities provided that you have 'the knowledge and skills to undertake this aspect of care and that (you) are adequately supervised as required' (NMC, 2007, p. 4). Your ability to contribute to record-keeping will be assessed in your practice area by the person delegating the responsibility for record-keeping to you (usually your mentor) – if they feel you are not competent they must clearly countersign any entries made by you. The NMC states this in its *Guidelines for records and record-keeping*:

> Record-keeping is an integral part of nursing, midwifery and specialist community public health nursing practice. It is a tool of professional practice and one that should help the care process. It is not separate from this process and it is not an optional extra to be fitted in if circumstances allow.
>
> (NMC, 2007, p. 1)

The NMC (2007, p.1) further says that good record-keeping helps to protect the welfare of patients/clients by promoting:

- high standards of clinical care;
- continuity of care;
- better communication and dissemination of information between members of the inter-professional health care team;
- an accurate account of treatment and care planning and delivery;

- the ability to identify problems, such as changes in the patient/client's condition, at any stage;
- the concept of confidentiality.

Patients and clients should be equal partners, whenever possible, in their completion of their records (NMC, 2007, p. 3). They have the right to expect that all health care professionals, including registered nurses and student nurses who contribute to their records, will practise a high standard of record-keeping (NMC, 2007, p. 1). Therefore, failure on the part of a registered nurse to maintain reasonable standards of record-keeping could be evidence of professional misconduct and subject to Fitness to Practice proceedings. Records can also be called as evidence by the Health Services Commissioner, before a court of law, or in a local investigation of a complaint made by a patient. This may include anything that makes reference to a patient (for example, care plans, diaries, etc.), and any absence of a record may be seen as a lack of care, negligence, inability to write a record, disinterest, concealment or a general failure to communicate in the best interests of the patient. A coroner recently stated: 'Nurses are good observers – it's only a question of whether or not they write their observations down – when they come to court to testify, facts which seemed trivial at the time take on a paramount importance' (anon).

Nurses have both a legal and professional duty of care; therefore their record-keeping should be able to demonstrate (NMC, 2007, p. 3):

- a full account of their assessment and the care that has been planned and provided;
- relevant information about the condition of the patient/client at any given time;
- the measures taken by the registered nurse and/or student nurse to respond to their needs;
- evidence that the registrant has understood and honoured their duty of care, that all reasonable steps have been taken to care for the patient/client and that any actions or omissions on the part of the registrant have not compromised their safety in any way;
- a record of any arrangements that have been made for the continuing care of a patient/client.

Therefore, all nurses should be familiar with the NMC guidelines, which can be accessed at **www.nmc-uk.org**. The salient points of these guidelines are listed below.

Content and style (NMC, 2007, p. 2)

There are a number of factors that contribute to effective record-keeping. Patient/client records should:

- be factual, consistent and accurate, written in such a way that the meaning is clear;
- be recorded as soon as possible after the event has occurred, providing current information on the care and condition of the patient/client;
- be recorded clearly and in such a manner that the text cannot be erased or deleted without a record of change;
- be recorded in such a manner that any justifiable alterations or additions are dated, timed and signed or clearly attributed to a named person in an identifiable role in such a way that the original entry can still be read clearly;
- be accurately dated, timed and signed, with the signature printed alongside the first entry where this is a written record, and attributed to a named person in an identifiable role for electronic records;
- not include abbreviations, jargon, meaningless phrases, irrelevant speculation and offensive subjective statements;
- be readable on any photocopies.

In addition, records should:

- be recorded, wherever possible, with the involvement of the patient/client or their carer;
- be written in terms that the patient/client can understand;
- be consecutive;
- identify risks and/or problems that have arisen and the action taken to rectify them;
- provide clear evidence of the care planned, the decisions made, the care delivered and the information shared.

MAINTAINING PROFESSIONAL KNOWLEDGE AND COMPETENCE

Once you are a registered nurse you will have to undertake post-registration education and practice (Prep). This is a set of NMC professional standards and guidance designed to help nurses provide the best possible care for patients and keep up to date with developments in practice by thinking and reflecting on their practice (NMC, 2008c).

In order to renew registration, registered nurses must provide a signed Notification of Practice (NOP), which asks them, among other things, to declare that they have met the Prep requirements. There are two separate Prep standards that affect registration (NMC, 2008c, p. 4).

- **The Prep (practice) standard** – nurses must have worked in some capacity by virtue of their nursing or midwifery qualification for a minimum of 450 hours during the previous three years, or have successfully undertaken an approved return to practice course within the last three years.
- **The Prep (continuing professional development) standard** – nurses must have undertaken and recorded their continuing professional development (CPD) over the three years prior to the renewal of their registration.

Continuing professional development is defined as:

> A process of lifelong learning for all individuals which meets the needs of patients and delivers health outcomes and health care priorities of the NHS which enables professionals to expand and fulfil their potential (HSC, 1999/194),

Although this definition specifically states NHS, it is applicable to all areas where registered nurses are employed.

To satisfy the Prep CPD standard (NMC, 2008c, p. 9), registered nurses must produce evidence that they:

- have undertaken at least 35 hours of learning activity relevant to their practice during the three years prior to renewal of registration;
- have maintained a personal professional profile (PPP) of their learning activity;
- comply with any request from the NMC to audit the way in which these requirements have been met.

Further information

For further details on how to meet the Prep requirements see *The Prep Handbook* (2008) at **www.nmc-uk.org**

COMMON REASONS WHY NURSES ARE REMOVED FROM THE REGISTER

Listed below are some of the common reasons why registered nurses are removed from the NMC register. Removal from the register is a result of findings of the Fitness to Practice panels where registered nurses' conduct and performance are measured against *The Code*. Anyone has the right to complain to the NMC about a registered nurse – fellow registered nurses, colleagues in other health care professions, patients and their families, employers, managers and the police (NMC, 2004) on the grounds of:

- failure to provide adequate care;
- failure to protect/promote the interest of patients;
- deliberately concealing unsafe practice;
- failure to act, knowing that a colleague or subordinate is improperly treating or abusing patients;
- committing criminal offences;
- failure to keep proper records, falsifying records;
- continued lack of competence despite opportunities to improve;
- physical or verbal abuse of patients;
- failure to administer medicines safely;
- theft from patients or employers;
- drug-related offences;
- alcohol or drug dependence;
- untreated serious mental illness;
- sexual abuse of patients;
- breach of confidentiality.

Perhaps on not such a serious scale, if you as a student nurse have any doubts about the actions or performance of a registered nurse, the NMC (2005) say you mustn't ignore the situation, although it could put you in a difficult position. They advise that you challenge the registered nurse as it may help them improve their practice.

Activity

Visit the NMC website at **www.nmc-uk.org/aArticle.aspx? ArticleID=191** and find details of recent Fitness to Practice cases that are reported there. Look at the facts of the cases and see how the NMC decided to deal with the allegations.

SUMMARY

Each registered nurse must ensure that they fulfil their duties according to the approved standards of practice expected of them. If something goes wrong they are accountable in the criminal courts, the civil courts, before their employer and before the Fitness to Practice Committees of the NMC for their activities, and would have to show that they had followed the approved accepted practice (Dimond, 2005). As a student nurse you have similar responsibilities to fulfil your duties, as registered nurses do, in all areas of practice.

Further reading

British Medical Association **www.bma.org.uk**
European Court of Human Rights **www.echr.coe.int**
General Medical Council **www.gmc-uk.org**
Health Service Ombudsman **www.ombudsman.org.uk**
Information Commission **www.dataprotection.gov.uk**
Law Society for England and Wales (has a useful section on clinical
    negligence) **www.lawsociety.org.uk**
Royal College of Nursing **www.rcn.org.uk**

REFERENCES

Banks, S. (2004) *Ethics, Accountability and the Social Professions.* Basingstoke: Palgrave

Burnard, P. and Chapman, C. (2003) *Professional and Ethical Issues In Nursing* (3rd edn). London: Ballière Tindall

Castledine, G. (1991) 'Accountability in delivering care'. *Nursing Standard*, 5 (25), 13: 28–30

Caulfield, H. (2005) *Vital Notes for Nurses: Accountability.* Oxford: Blackwell

Department of Health (1999) *Caldicott Guardians*, NHS Executive, HSC, 1999/012. London: Department Of Health

Department of Health (2001) *Reference Guide to Consent for Examination or Treatment.* London: Department Of Health

Dimond, B. (2005) *Legal Aspects Of Nursing* (4th edn). London: Pearson Longman

HSC (1999/194) *Continuing Professional Development (Quality In The New NHS).* London: Department Of Health

National Council for Palliative Care. *Guidance to the Mental Capacity Act 2005*. **www.ncpc.org.uk** (accessed Oct 2008)

Nursing and Midwifery Council (2004) *Complaints About Unfitness to Practice: A guide for members of the public*. London: NMC

Nursing and Midwifery Council (2005) An *NMC Guide for Students of Nursing and Midwifery*. London: NMC

Nursing and Midwifery Council (2007) *NMC Record Keeping Guidance*. London: NMC

Nursing and Midwifery Council (2008a) *The Code: Standards For Conduct, Performance and Ethics For Nurses and Midwives*. London: NMC

Nursing and Midwifery Council (2008b) *What We Mean by Good Health and Good Character*. **www.nmc-uk.org** (accessed October 2008)

Nursing and Midwifery Council (2008c) *The Prep Handbook*. London: NMC

Nursing and Midwifery Council (2008d) *Advice Sheet: Providing care in an emergency situation outside the workplace*. London: NMC

Peate, I. (2006) *Becoming a Nurse in The 21st Century*. Chichester: Wiley

Richards, A. and Edwards, S. (2008) *A Nurse's Survival Guide to the Ward*. London: Churchill Livingstone

Tingle, J. and Cribb, A. (2006) *Nursing Law and Ethics*. Oxford: Blackwell

Useful websites

Department of Constitutional Affairs **www.dca.gov.uk** (Mental Capacity Act)

Department of Health **www.dh.gov.uk**

Nursing and Midwifery Council **www.nmc-uk.org**

Chapter 5

Values and Health Care Ethics

The purpose of this chapter is to outline the theories and principles used in the health care ethics and values debate, but remember that any amount of reading will not equip you with a set of absolute rules to solve all the moral problems you encounter. Tschudin (2003) believes ethics can only be described in terms of principles and never in terms of absolutes, while Aristotle is reputed to have said that 'there is a solution to every problem – the only problem is finding it!'

Outcomes

On completion of this chapter you should be able to:

- explore the concept of values and patients' rights in nursing;
- briefly describe the ethical theories of deontology and utilitarianism;
- briefly describe the four principles of health care ethics (in respect of autonomy, beneficence, non-maleficence and justice).

VALUES AND RIGHTS

Values are a fundamental component of the provision, practice and delivery of health and social care . . . they are particular kinds of beliefs concerned with the worth of an idea or behaviour and are important in guiding actions, judgments, behaviour and attitudes towards others. In addition they are concerned with the norms, rules, habits, expectations and assumptions that are at the heart of society and form the basis of social interactions and relationships.

(Cuthbert and Quallington, 2008, p. 1)

The term 'values' is often linked with the term 'ethics', which, in turn, is often used with the term 'morals'. According to Beauchamp and Childress (2001, p. 5), morality refers to 'social conventions about right and wrong human conduct, whereas ethics is a general term referring to both morality and ethical theory'. All these terms will be discussed in the following pages.

Values are personal beliefs that influence how you act and how you judge others' actions. Development of your personal moral 'knowledge' and values comes from a variety of sources: your upbringing, gender, class, age, religious/spiritual beliefs, peer groups, culture, education, life experiences – the list could be endless, but the important factor is that all perspectives are personal to you and often change as you progress through life.

Every one of us is influenced by our value system. Values have the potential to motivate and guide our choices and decision-making abilities (Peate, 2007), but personal and professional values may not always be the same and may differ from those of another nurse, even though you are caring for the same patients. This is because values are personal. For example, Cuthbert and Quallington (2008) give the analogy of two nurses working on a maternity ward who have very different views on abortion, but are required to deliver the same professional care.

According to Hope (2004, cited in Peate, 2007, p. 48), most of us have 'gut reactions' to what we think is morally right or wrong in certain situations. However, there are some viewpoints that most of us take into account when evaluating others' actions and behaviour, particularly in professional circumstances and regardless of our personal opinions.

- **Legal** – actions are right if they comply with the law, wrong if they do not.
- **Professional** – actions are right if they are supported by codes of professional conduct, protocols and evidence-based practice, wrong if they do not.
- **Religious beliefs** – how does God or religious teaching view the action?
- **Social convention** – does the action conform to acceptable norms of behaviour in society?
- **Practical** – an action is right if it is the easiest and most practical way to achieve the desired aim or intention. Conflict will arise if the action goes against any of the above or harms the patient.

Fry and Johnstone (2002, cited in Peate, 2007) point out that nurses should remember that, just as you have your own set of personal values, so do patients and there could be a potential conflict. In this case they advise that nurses must respect the values of others, but ensure that a balance is achieved in relation to the patient's rights and their own professional duties.

Patients' rights

Patients' rights are sometimes referred to as 'entitlements' or 'claims' and stem from the premise that individuals are unique and valuable and therefore should be afforded certain rights. These are sometimes described as 'positive rights' and 'negative rights'. Positive rights require society, or another individual, to do something positive in order to fulfil or uphold human and legal rights – for example, health care can only be realised if society ensures that health care systems exist and that the individuals in the system fulfil their duty to provide care. A negative right, sometimes referred to as a 'qualified right', relates to the freedom to do something without interference – for example, the freedom of expression and freedom to practise one's preferred religion (or not practise a religion) (Cuthbert and Quallington, 2008).

Human rights (see also Chapter 6 on 'The UK as a culturally-diverse society')

The major piece of international legislation relating to rights is the Human Rights Act 1998. This Act sets out what each person has a right to expect with regard to fundamental human rights and freedoms regardless of gender, disability, ethnic identity, sexuality or class. It makes it unlawful for public authorities (and therefore nurses) to act in a way which is incompatible with the various articles within the Act.

Within the 14 articles of the Human Rights Act, McHale and Gallagher (2003) differentiate between absolute rights, limited rights and qualified rights. Absolute rights cannot be restricted – for example, Article 2, 'The right to life', and Article 3, 'Prohibition of torture' (in this regard consider the treatment of inmates at Guantanamo Bay). Limited rights include such articles as Article 5, 'Right to liberty and security', that contains a series of legitimate exceptions like, for example, the lawful detention of persons for the prevention of spreading of infectious diseases, persons of unsound mind, alcoholics or drug addicts or vagrants. McHale and Gallagher (2003) also refer to a third group, which they call qualified rights, that are found in Articles 8, 9 and 10 – 'Right to respect for private and family life', 'Freedom of thought, conscience and religion' and

'Freedom of expression' respectively. These fall into the same category as Cuthbert and Quallington's 'negative rights'. The most pertinent of the 14 articles to nursing are the following.

- **Article 8: Right to respect for private and family life, home and correspondence.** This confers the right for each person to live their own life as is reasonable within a democratic society and takes account of the freedoms and rights of others. This right can also include the right to have information about the person such as, for example, official records including medical information, kept private and confidential. It also places restrictions on the extent to which any public authority can invade an individual's privacy about their body without their permission. In the health care context this has implications in relation to decisions of consent and refusal of treatment, and confidentiality of patient records.
- **Article 9: Freedom of thought, conscience and religion.** This provides an absolute right for a person to hold the thoughts, positions of conscience or religion of their choice. This includes the right for the person to practise or demonstrate their religion in private or public (as long as it does not interfere with the rights and freedoms of others). In a health care setting this article is particularly applicable in relation to the right of the health care professionals to opt out of certain procedures on the basis of conscientious objection such as, for example, assisting with pregnancy terminations. Equally it applies to patients who refuse treatment on religious grounds like, for example, Jehovah's Witnesses and the transfusion of blood.
- **Article 14: Freedom from discrimination.** In the context of the Act, discrimination is defined as 'treating people in similar situations differently, or those in different situations in the same way, without proper justification' (DCA, 2006, p. 25). Among other issues this includes associated sex and sexual orientation, age, race, colour, language, religion, disability, political or other opinion, national or social origin, association with a national minority, property, birth (for example, whether born inside or outside of marriage) and marital status. Regardless of status everyone is entitled to equal access to all the rights set out in the Act.

www.opsi.gov.uk/acts

Legal rights

These are rights that have to be afforded to patients due to laws of the land (see Chapter 4 on 'Legal and professional issues'). They include criminal acts such as murder, manslaughter, rape, theft, etc. (all of which nurses have been found guilty of), and civil cases where an action for negligence results from a breach of duty of care.

Professional considerations

These are clauses within codes of practice and standards that professionals have to adhere to, to maintain their 'registration'. The NMC states that one of their primary functions is to protect the public, and inform the public of the standards of professional conduct they can expect of a registered practitioner (**www.nmc-uk.org**). It is for this reason that any member of the public can access the NMC website and read the various standards and guidelines that indicate how they should be treated. In addition to the NMC *Code* (2008), there are various standards published by both the NMC and the Department of Health concerning issues such as confidentiality, consent, delivering competent care, advocacy and anti-discriminatory practice – all outlining patients' rights in these respects, and the need for nurses to respect their contents. Other publications have statements about privacy, dignity and respect implicit within them – for example, National Service Frameworks, NICE guidelines and the Mental Capacity Act.

The Department of Health recently issued the *NHS Constitution* (Department of Health, 2009), which establishes the principles and values of the NHS in England. It sets out:

> the rights to which patients, public and staff are entitled and pledges which the NHS is committed to achieve, together with responsibilities which the public, patients and staff owe to one another to ensure that the NHS operates fairly and effectively. All NHS bodies and private and third sector providers supplying NHS services will be required by law to take account of this Constitution in their decisions and actions.
>
> (Department of Health, 2009, p. 2)

Respect, dignity and privacy

The concepts of privacy, dignity and respect can be found in many health care professionals' codes of practice. Indeed, the first clause of the NMC *Code* states: 'Make the care of patients your first concern, treating them as individuals and respecting their dignity' (NMC, 2008, p. 2). In terms of 'respect for a person' the words 'dignity' and 'respect' are often used interchangeably, in that dignity means being worthy of respect, and that giving a person respect will maintain their dignity. Cuthbert and Quallington (2008) believe nurses should respect everyone as a valued unique individual, and cite Dillon (1992) as saying respect in care involves:

- a belief in the value of persons as individuals and as members of society;
- treating people in the manner in which you expect to be treated;
- showing consideration for another person's feelings and interests;
- an attitude demonstrating that you value another person.

Respect is shown in many ways – demonstrating a genuine interest in your patients, listening to them, preserving their modesty, addressing the patient by the name they prefer, etc. However, there are other forms of respect that nurses have to acknowledge – 'respect for boundaries' such as the laws associated with consent, confidentiality and within codes of conduct, and 'respect for authority' that you should show to personnel more senior to you.

Physical privacy can be hard to promote in a health care situation, and yet patients may be at their most vulnerable away from their familiar surroundings and yearn for privacy. Many environments do not lend themselves to privacy and it can be a challenge to promote (for example, mixed-sex wards, bedpans behind curtains, personal hygiene needs, etc.). However, treating the patient with dignity and respect at these times can go a long way to enhancing care where privacy may be compromised. It should be remembered that privacy is also extended to the patient's space and belongings. In their own environment this is relatively easy for them to control but in a health care setting they are often unable to limit the power of others to intrude.

Dignity and privacy are part of the benchmarks published by the Department of Health (2001) when they introduced *Essence of Care.* This is a set of guidelines aimed at promoting good person-centred care organised around 'factors' and 'benchmarks'.

Care Quality Commission

To ensure that these guidelines, and indeed all Department of Health guidelines and standards, are upheld, the government introduced the Care Quality Commission in April 2009. This body is the independent regulator of health and social care in England, and its aim is to make sure better care is provided for everyone, whether in hospital, care homes, people's own homes, or elsewhere. In doing this they regulate health and adult social care services provided by the NHS, local authorities, private companies and voluntary organisations (see Chapter 7 on 'Quality assurance').

Factor	Benchmark
1. Attitudes and behaviours.	Patients feel that they matter all of the time.
2. Personal world and personal identity.	Patients experience care in an environment that actively encompasses individual values, beliefs and personal relationships.
3. Personal boundaries and space.	Patients' personal space is actively promoted by all staff.
4. Communicating with staff and patients.	Communication between staff and patients takes place in a manner that respects their individuality.
5. Privacy of patient – confidentiality of patient information.	Patient information is shared to enable care, with their consent.
6. Privacy, dignity and modesty.	Patients' care actively promotes their privacy and dignity, and protects their modesty.
7. Availability of an area for complete privacy.	Patients and/or carers can access an area that safely provides privacy.
Privacy = Freedom from intrusion *Dignity* = Being worthy of respect	

(Department of Health, 2001, p.120)

Figure 1: *Essence of Care* benchmarks

Activity

How would you ensure that: 'Patients experience care in an environment that actively encompasses individual values, beliefs and personal relationships' (benchmark 2)? Make brief notes.

HEALTH CARE ETHICS (adapted from Ian Donaldson)

As stated earlier, it is important to recognise that every individual will have differing opinions and views, and sometimes there are no right or wrong attitudes or beliefs. Burnard and Kendrick (1998) note that the term 'ethics' is notoriously ambiguous, conjuring up different images for different people. However, everyone should be able to express their views, while remembering not to exclude alternative viewpoints. Ethical debate is about individuals reflecting on their own and others' viewpoints with insight and reasoning.

Nurses are often confronted with moral dilemmas – this is when they recognise that they both ought and ought not to perform a particular action as there are equally compelling reasons for and against it. This is made increasingly difficult when nurses have differing views and values, often causing disagreements either between colleagues or patients. Griffith and Tengnah (2008) give the example of a nurse who believes a doctor's decision not to resuscitate a patient with a terminal illness is wrong – the nurse believes the patient's life should be sustained, and is suddenly faced with a dilemma about what is right or wrong. Both decisions are lawful, so the decision is one of morality. Another good example of this can be found in the constant debate over abortion – whose rights prevail?

Using theories and principles may help to guide moral deliberations. There are a wide range of differing moral standpoints but three particular ways of moral reasoning have been extremely influential in the shaping and discussions of health care ethics. They are the theories of utilitarianism, deontology and the principles of health care ethics.

Utilitarianism

This idea was first put forward by Bentham in the eighteenth century and refined by John Stuart Mill in the nineteenth century. Mill believed that the way to evaluate what was morally right or wrong was to examine the outcome or 'consequences' of that action – i.e. producing good consequences, not just having good intentions. Mill's golden rule was that actions are right if they promote happiness and wrong if they produce the reverse of happiness. This rule is often abbreviated to 'the greatest happiness or the greatest good to the greatest number' and that 'the end (the consequences) justifies the means (the action taken)'.

An argument against utilitarianism is that it can promote activities that are a selfish pursuit of pleasures at the expense of everyone else. Mill attempted to solve this critique with two additional 'rules'. He said that actions were good if they created the greatest amount of happiness. This argument means that selfish activities that create happiness for one person but unhappiness in a great number of other people are not acceptable (consider how this 'rule' prevents a paedophile from justifying his activities). Mill's second 'rule' was to say that there is a difference between the quantity and quality of pleasures that cause happiness. He believed that it is better to pursue high-quality pleasures, which he describes as intellectual, aesthetic and imaginative, rather than lower-quality pleasures, which he describes as 'mere animal instincts'. However, a major critique of utilitarianism is that one cannot be certain of predicting consequences and, as such, utilitarianism is not useful to guide individuals as to what they ought to do.

Included in the definition of utilitarianism is the criterion of the 'rightness or wrongness of an action' and whether it is useful in furthering the goal of the greatest happiness for the greatest number (Thompson, *et al.*, 2006). This can have implications for truth-telling – as a nurse you would have to weigh up the consequences as to whether telling the truth would lead to more happiness than unhappiness. In this instance, even if a decision is made to tell the truth in order to arrive at the greatest good for the greatest number, this may not be morally correct, and a deontological approach may be more appropriate (Peate, 2007).

Deontology

The theory of deontology was put forward by Kant in the eighteenth century. He believed it is the 'action' that is important and not the consequences. Kant was also concerned with the motive and intentions of the individual performing the action, and argued that the action is only morally right if the individual is motivated by goodwill. Kant's theory is often called the dutiful view of morality, where we are bound by duty to act in a particular way, and not to produce certain consequences.

You may consider that there are certain actions, such as being honest, telling the truth and keeping a promise, that are right and good actions, but how can an individual decide where their duty lies? Kant argued that we know where our duty lies by considering this question: 'Do I want everyone to behave as I am proposing to do in these circumstances?' This he called the 'categorical imperative, or a universal law'. An example of this could be to 'always keep a promise' because you would want others to keep their promises to you, so it is therefore something that you would want to be a universal law.

Kant's theory of deontology is criticised for the problems it can create when a categorical imperative, such as always telling the truth, is followed in every situation. However, this criticism seems to miss the point on two counts – firstly, for many the idea that certain actions are right in themselves and ought to be followed is an important part of their view of morality; secondly, it ignores the process by which the truth is told.

It is important to stress that while both these theories of utilitarianism (concerned with the outcome) and deontology (concerned with the motive) are different, they do not always lead to different evaluations of a particular action.

Principles of health care ethics

Beauchamp and Childress wrote their very influential book on bio-medical ethics in the late 1970s, (various editions have been produced since) and many nurses refer to this text. The authors suggest that there are four key principles in health care ethics and argue that by examining a dilemma using these principles the nurse will be helped to decide what the right course of action is. The key principles are:

- respect for Autonomy;
- Beneficence;
- Non-Maleficence;
- Justice.

Autonomy

Autonomy, additionally referred to as self-determination or self-rule or simply 'being one's own person', is defined as 'the capacity to think, decide and act on the basis of such thought and decision . . . freely and independently without let or hindrance' (Gillon, 1985, p. 6). Autonomy is seen as being increasingly important within health care, and is closely allied to respect for people's choices. Cuthbert and Quallington (2008, p. 59) suggest that definitions of autonomy often include references to such terms as:

- self-governance;
- independence;
- individuality;
- self-choice/individual choice;
- freedom/freedom of will;
- being one's own person.

Autonomy is linked with many issues in nursing including values, respect and privacy. In terms of values, Beauchamp and Childress (2001) suggest respect for autonomy is based on the general recognition that an individual has unconditional worth with the capacity to determine their own destiny. Dworkin (1988) believes that people know what is best for them, so giving them the right to express their autonomy will contribute to their happiness and well-being.

Patients' autonomy can be compromised when they enter a health care setting. What had previously been everyday decisions can be taken away from them – what to wear, when to shower, when (and what) to eat, where and when they sleep. Peate (2007) points out that working things out with the patient and their family can ensure that as much autonomous decision-making as possible is retained by the patient, and is a key aspect of the nurse's role. Thompson *et al.* (2006) further suggest nurses should actually protect patients who suffer loss of autonomy through illness, injury or mental disorder. Ramsay (1970) states that autonomy is about working to maintain the optimum degree of independence for the patient and sharing knowledge, care and skills in such as way as to empower the patient, thereby avoiding creating and perpetuating dependency. This, in essence, is allowing the patient freedom to make their own decisions and express their personal preferences and aspirations.

The NMC *Code* (2008) upholds the patient's right to autonomy in many ways – it advocates confidentiality, consent, privacy and dignity among other important issues concerned with autonomy. Dworkin (1988) considers these (particularly consent) when he states the patient's autonomy depends on conditions such as:

- the ability to make independent choices;
- adequate information;
- adequate knowledge.

For example, it is well recognised in this country that any mentally competent adult (the law relating to children giving consent is different) has the right in law to consent to any touching of his or her person. For an individual to give consent, and so exercise their autonomy, it is clear that information is required to enable an informed decision to be made.

Activity

How free are you to make choices? To what extent are you an autonomous person? Think of the last time you made a choice – did you really have total autonomy or were there things which stood in the way? (From Peate, 2007, p. 54).

Paternalism

When an individual acts to override someone's autonomy by restricting information or choices, it is described as paternalism. This is done with the intent of benefiting that person but it takes away their choice (i.e. a doctor advocating surgery when the patient does not want an operation). It is always very difficult to know what the right course of action is to take in this type of situation. A guideline could be to remember that respect for autonomy is of central importance when considering a patient's request, and asking yourself two questions. Firstly, 'is the patient mentally competent?' in any situation where a patient's capacity to make an informed decision will compromise their autonomy. Secondly, 'does the consideration rest on whether one of the other principles (beneficence, non-maleficence or justice) carries greater weight in the particular situation?' It is also useful to refer the NMC *Code* (2008), which is very clear about the nurse's role in gaining consent.

Beneficence

Beneficence is the duty to do good and avoid doing harm to others (both physically and psychologically), and has been described as 'do unto others as you would have them do unto you' (Thompson *et al.*, 2006). As a nurse you have a duty of care to your patients (NMC, 2008) and a duty to promote what is best for your patients. This has been the guiding principle in health care for some time, and is utilised by acting in the patient's 'best interests'.

However, acting in the patient's best interests raises the question of who should be the judge of what is best for the patient (Hope, 2004). Linked with the principle of autonomy, it should be the patient who decides but, in some instances, this is not possible. The Mental Capacity Act 2005 recognises this and is concerned with protecting those who lack the capacity to make their own decisions or consent to treatment in a variety of health and social circumstances – this can either be on a temporary or permanent basis (see Chapter 4 on 'Legal and professional issues'). The

NMC (2008, p. 4) highlights this when talking about temporary inability to make decisions in *The Code*: 'You must be able to demonstrate that you have acted in someone's best interests if you have provided care in an emergency'.

The principle of beneficence can cause tensions if a competent patient decides on an action that is not in their best interests (for example, a Jehovah's Witness refusing a life-saving blood transfusion) where, if action was taken, the hospital staff would be 'violating the bodily integrity of the person without consent' (Hope, 2004), and which, in legal terms, would amount to committing battery.

Seedhouse (2009) includes truth-telling in his discussion of beneficence, and believes it is a central principle of conduct. However, he also believes there are some instances when it is better not to tell the truth, thereby propounding the principle of non-maleficence. He gives the example of allowing patients to read their medical records. Truth-telling relates closely to respect for the person and their autonomy, particularly when it comes down to the giving of information on which people will base their choices and decisions in health and care (Cuthbert and Quallington, 2008). Indeed the NMC (2008) states that patients are entitled to accurate and 'truthful' information, which is presented in a way they can understand.

Activity

Consider a situation from your placements when information was withheld.

- Was this justified? What ethical, legal and professional implications arose from this type of action?
- How was the situation resolved?
- Do you think this was satisfactory – if not, why not?

Non-maleficence

This principle states 'above all to do no harm', which has been likened to the reverse of beneficence, but it is not quite the same thing as many nursing interventions do cause harm. However, it is clear that to intentionally cause distress is morally wrong. Beauchamp and Childress (2001) point out that obligations not to harm are sometimes more stringent than obligations to help, and the NMC endorses this in *The*

Code (2008) when it states that in caring for patients nurses must provide a safe standard of care that avoids or minimises risks (NMC, 2008). Apart from the ethical aspects of this, failure to comply could bring a court action for negligence.

Activity

Can you think of a situation where harm could be caused to a patient but, in the long term, it would be in their best interests?

Justice

The final principle to consider is that of justice – that 'everyone is valued equally and treated alike' (Peate, 2007, p. 57). According to Hope (2004, p. 66), there are four elements to this principle.

- **Distributive justice** (sometimes termed entitlement): Patients in similar situations should normally have access to the same health care and, in determining what level of health care should be available for one set of patients, account should be taken of the effect of such a use of resources on other patients. In other words, limited resources should be distributed fairly.
- **Respect for the law**: The fact that some act is, or is not, within the law is of moral relevance. Some people may take the view that it might be, in some situations, morally right to break the law, but laws are made through a democratic process and have to be enforced.
- **Rights**: The fundamental idea that a person has rights is a safeguard to their rights being respected, even if overall the social good is thereby diminished.
- **Retributive justice**: This concerns the fitting of punishment to the crime – an element not really concerned with health care provision.

When considering distributive justice or 'entitlement', there is a range of different options for the allocation of resources in health care, including:

- equal share to everyone;
- random distribution;
- on a first come, first served basis;
- according to need;

- to deserving cases;
- to treat as many as possible.

Some of these options can in themselves create inequalities. For example, to allocate an equal share of a resource to everyone may in some cases be perceived as wrong because some individuals are disadvantaged as they have a greater need.

Further reading

Cuthbert, S. and Quallington, J. (2008) *Values for Care Practice*. Exeter: Reflect Press, provides a detailed exploration of health care values.

REFERENCES

Beauchamp, T. and Childress, J. (2001) *Principles of Bio-medical Ethics.* Oxford: Oxford University Press

Burnard, P. and Kendrick, K. (1998) *Ethical Counselling: A workbook for nurses*. London: Edward Arnold

Cuthbert, S. and Quallington, J. (2008) *Values for Care Practice*. Exeter: Reflect Press

Department for Constitutional Affairs (2006) *A Guide to the Human Rights Act 1998* (3rd edn). London: DCA

Department of Health (2001) *Essence of Care: Patient-focused benchmarking for health care practitioners*. London: HMSO

Department of Health (2005) *The Mental Capacity Act*. London: HMSO

Department of Health (2009) *The NHS Constitution*. London: Department of Health

Dillon, R. (1992) 'Respect and care: Toward moral integration'. *Canadian Journal of Philosophy*, 22: 105–32, in Cuthbert, S. and Quallington, J. (2008) *Values for Care Practice*. Exeter: Reflect Press

Dworkin, G. (1988) *The Theory and Practice of Autonomy*. New York: Cambridge University Press

Fry, S. and Johnstone, M. (2002) *Ethics in Nursing Practice: A guide to ethical decision making*. Oxford: Blackwell, in Peate, I. (2007) *Becoming a Nurse in the 21st Century*. Chichester: Wiley

Gillon, R. (1985) *Philosophical Medical Ethics*. Chichester: Wiley

Griffith, R. and Tengnah, C. (2008) *Law and Professional Issues in Nursing*. Exeter: Learning Matters

Hope, T. (2004) *Medical Ethics: A very short introduction.* Oxford: University Press

McHale, J. and Gallagher, A. (2003) *Nursing and Human Rights.* Edinburgh: Butterworth Heinemann

Nursing and Midwifery Council (2008) *The Code: Standards of conduct, performance and ethics for nurses and midwives.* London: NMC

Peate, I. (2007) *Becoming a Nurse in the 21st Century.* Chichester: Wiley

Ramsay, P. (1970) *The Patient as Person.* New Haven: Yale University Press

Seedhouse, D. (2009) *The Heart of Healthcare.* Chichester: Wiley

Thompson, I., Melia, K., Boyd, K. and Horsburgh, D. (2006) *Nursing Ethics* (5th edn). Edinburgh: Churchill Livingstone

Tschudin, V. (2003) *Ethics in Nursing: The caring relationship.* London: Butterworth Heinemann

Useful websites

www.nmc-uk.org (accessed March 2009)
www.opsi.gov.uk/acts (accessed March 2009)

Chapter 6

The UK as a Culturally Diverse Society

The aim of this chapter is to briefly explore the concept of culture and raise your awareness regarding the delivery of health care within a multicultural society.

Outcomes

On completion of this chapter you should be able to:

- briefly discuss the concept of culture and associated terminology;

- appraise the customs and factors that may impact upon the provision, delivery and receipt of health care for some service users;

- reflect on your own personal experiences of the multicultural dimensions of care;

- outline key issues associated with transcultural care;

- outline current legislation important to practice.

INTRODUCTION

The population of Britain at the beginning of the twenty-first century, like many European countries, has been shaped considerably by post-war patterns of emigration and immigration. According to the last Office of Population Censuses and Surveys (2001) there were approximately 4.5 million people of differing ethnic origin residing in the United Kingdom, constituting 7.9 per cent of the population. People from India were identified as the largest of these groups, followed by those from Pakistan, those of mixed ethnic backgrounds, black Caribbean, black African and then people from Bangladesh. Given these statistics it is easy to understand why the UK is considered to be a multicultural, multiethnic, and multifaith society.

CULTURE

According to Macionis and Plummer (2005, p. 106), culture encompasses 'the values, beliefs, behaviour, practices and material objects that constitute a people's way of life'. It includes such factors as how people dress, their marriage customs and family life, their patterns of work, religious ceremonies and leisure pursuits. It is also perceived as a bridge to the past as well as a guide to the future. A review of the literature, for example Papadopoulos (2006), Andrews and Boyle (2007) and Jirwe (2008), suggest there are four main characteristics of culture:

1 **It is learned** from birth through the process of language acquisition and socialisation. From society's point of view, socialisation is the way culture is transmitted and the individual is fitted into the group's organised way of life.
2 **It is shared** by all members of the same cultural group; in fact it is the sharing of cultural beliefs and patterns that binds people together under one identity as a group (even though this is not always a conscious process).
3 **It is an adaptation** to specific activities related to environmental and technical factors and to the availability of natural resources.
4 **It is a dynamic, ever-changing process**. People do not merely receive their culture from others, they also make it and remake it continually in a process of interaction with others.

Hofstede and Hofstede (2004) also identify numerous layers of culture that include:

- national;
- regional;
- gender;
- generational;
- professional;
- organisational;
- social class.

Finally, Geiger and Davidhizar (2007) suggest the following cultural phenomena exist.

- **Communication** – there is no known culture without a grammatically complex language, with different languages having different meanings.
- **Social organisation** – family systems and religious and other organisational groups vary among cultures.
- **Space** – various cultures have different concepts about social, personal space and territory.
- **Time** – each culture has its own conception and orientation of time.
- **Environmental control** – the values, beliefs and concepts of health practices vary widely among cultural groups – N.B. that because it is not always easy to understand the logic of a particular belief or practice, does not mean there is not one; it need not be logically based on the laws of Western medical science to be valid and practical.
- **Biological considerations** – constitutional endowment and vulnerability differ among people representing different cultures.

Associated cultural terminology

Terminology closely associated with the term 'culture' are those of ethnicity, ethnocentrism and race.

Ethnicity

There does not appear to be a single, universally accepted concept of ethnicity and this in itself can pose problems for nurses caring for patients/clients from diverse multiethnic groups. It is generally perceived as a term that represents a given social group with a shared history, sense of identity, country of origin, language, religion and cultural practices that characterise and distinguish them from other groups. Ethnic differences are wholly learnt and a result of socialisation and acculturation.

Ethnocentrism

According to Macionis and Plummer (2005 p. 119), this term refers to 'the practice of judging another culture by the standards of one's own culture', i.e. the assumption that one's own cultural group is superior to that of others. (N.B. to adopt such an approach would, obviously, be totally against providing holistic care to individual patients.)

Race

According to the Commission for Racial Equality (2007), the word 'race' once meant simply 'family'. Later it was used more loosely for national groups such as, for example, the French or German race. In the nineteenth century, scientists took it over to describe the 'races of man': groups defined by their physical appearance and different from one another in aspects such as skin colour, hair type and body shape, etc. Numerous theories were developed about these different races, which have now long since been discredited as unscientific and very wrong. Race is now widely acknowledged as a social/political construct rather than a biological or genetic fact.

However culture and associated terms are defined, it is important to remember that it has historic, present and future dimensions and has immense implications for the care you need to provide. Culture is not homogenous and therefore generalisations about individual members from a group should not be made as they can lead to stereotypical attitudes, cultural misunderstanding, prejudices and discrimination (Jirwe, 2008).

CULTURE IN PRACTICE

Given the population profile of the UK, you will inevitably find yourself in the position of caring for patients/clients from a variety of cultural/ethnic backgrounds, which will require you to have an understanding of the knowledge and skills required for effective transcultural nursing.

Activity

What do you think is meant by the term 'transcultural nursing'?

Leininger and McFarland (2002) suggest that transcultural nursing is theory and practice that focuses specifically on comparing the care for people with differences and similarities in beliefs, values and cultures in order to provide meaningful and beneficial health care. Wagner (2002) suggests that to achieve this requires both health care practitioners and the institution to consider how their practice can guarantee 'recognition, respect and nurturing' of the individual patient's cultural identity. Gerrish *et al.* (1996, cited in RCN, 2006) suggest this can involve the need to:

- reflect honestly on your own ethnicity;
- interrogate (both intellectually and emotionally) your response to the reality of ethnicity among your patient/client group;
- make explicit any implicit attitudes that might impact negatively on the care given to people of different ethnic backgrounds.

They also suggest that nursing professionals need to acquire and develop transcultural 'communicative competence'. Again, at the heart of this lies the capacity for 'adaptability in the sense that the practitioner is able to suspend or modify their own cultural expectations and accommodates new cultural demands . . .'. This requires the nurse to learn and understand the cultural values, behavioural patterns and interaction in specific cultures.

It is also worth remembering that the Nursing and Midwifery Council *Code* (2008) identifies that you must:

Make the care of people your first concern, treating them as individuals and respecting their dignity – you must not discriminate in any way against those in your care . . . (p. 2)

Be open and honest, act with integrity and uphold the reputation of your profession – you must demonstrate a personal and professional commitment to equality and diversity. (p. 9)

This means that every practitioner should seek to ensure that they provide and deliver care that meets the religious, dietary and linguistic requirements of patients, while ensuring that the principle of individualised care is not compromised.

The following brief notes seek to either remind you, or raise your awareness, with regard to some differing cultural/spiritual beliefs you may encounter while working as a nurse.

Christianity

Christians believe in the Holy Trinity of one God, the father of mankind, who created heaven and earth and who sent his son Jesus Christ to save mankind, and then sent the Holy Spirit to continue his work in human affairs. Christians believe that everything is created and given life by God the Father. Christianity stresses the importance of living a good life in response to God's love. It encompasses many groups and sects, but the main ones in the UK are the Anglican Church (which includes the Church of England, Church of Wales, Church of Scotland and Church of Ireland), the Roman Catholic Church, the free or nonconformist churches (for example the Baptist Church, Methodist Church) and the Eastern Orthodox Churches (for example the Greek and Russian Orthodox churches).

The Christian holy book is the Bible, the interpretation of which can differ between different sects or groups and so has implications for delivery and acceptance of treatment and care. It is therefore very important that you establish from the outset to which Christian sect or group an individual belongs.

Considerations for practice

Diet

Most Christians do not follow religious dietary restrictions, although some Roman Catholics may wish not to eat meat on Fridays, Ash Wednesday or Good Friday. They should therefore be offered a fish or vegetarian alternative.

Prayers

Some Christians may wish to receive Holy Communion and, possibly, the Anointing of the Sick, which involves being anointed with holy oil. A private and, where possible, quiet area of the care environment should be found if these rituals are taking place.

Dying and death

Roman Catholics may wish a priest to carry out the sacrament of the Last Rites or Extreme Unction (anointing). If they are able, the individual may also wish to receive Holy Communion and confess their sins to the priest either before receiving Holy Communion or separately. There are no particular rituals associated with last offices.

Jehovah's Witnesses

Jehovah's Witnesses consider their religion to be a restoration of original first-century Christianity. They accept both the Old and the New Testament of the Bible as inspired by God. They believe in one God, 'Jehovah', with the commands in the Bible being very important and they therefore try to live by them at all times.

Considerations for practice

Jehovah's Witnesses are totally opposed to taking blood or blood products into the body. This means that they will not accept blood transfusions even in life-threatening situations. However, they may accept alternative treatments.

Diet

Anything that contains blood or blood products is unacceptable, as is meat that has come from an animal that has been strangled, shot or not bled properly. If in doubt, Jehovah's Witnesses should be offered a vegetarian diet.

Patient confidentiality

Confidentiality must be maintained at all times and the patient's permission must be sought regarding what information they would like to be passed on to their family.

Death and dying

There are no particular rites and rituals associated with death and dying.

Hinduism

Largely confined to India, Hinduism is an amalgamation of many local faiths and is inextricably linked to culture and social structure. Hindus believe there is one God who can be worshipped and understood in many different forms. There is a belief in reincarnation in which the status and caste (hereditary or marital social class system) of each life is determined by the behaviour in the last life.

Hinduism does not have one leader, a unified code of conduct or creed. Because of this diversity it is difficult to generalise about what a specific individual might believe.

Considerations for practice

Physical examination

Generally, Hindu patients will have a strong preference for being treated and cared for by health care staff who are of the same gender. Privacy during any procedure is very important and female patients may be reluctant to remove clothing. They may also wish for a family member to act as a chaperone when physical examination and procedures are being carried out. Care must be taken not to remove any jewellery, threads, etc., without the patient's/family's permission as they often have a religious significance.

Personal hygiene

Hindus prefer to shower rather than bathe and should always be provided with water for washing when they go to the toilet.

Diet

Most Hindus are vegetarian, refusing to take the lives of animals for food. Devout Hindus would not eat off a plate on which meat has been served so an acceptable alternative (for example a plastic or paper plate) might need to be found.

Medication

Medication that contains animal products should be avoided.

Family and individual

As Hindus are intimately integrated with their extended family, there may be issues related to decision-making. Often decisions may be taken by a senior member of the family, or a female patient may wish her husband to consent to any treatment on her behalf.

Hindu patients tend to be visited frequently by their extended family, which can cause some difficulties with regard to preset visiting times and the 'numbers of visitors' policies that exist in most hospitals. The family may also wish to perform religious ceremonies with the patient. Privacy should be afforded to allow this to occur.

Prayer and ritual observance

Devout Hindus pray three times a day (at sunrise, noon and sunset). They should be assisted to wash prior to prayers if they are unable to do so independently. Where possible a quiet area should be provided and they should not be disturbed during prayer. Patients may wish to have statues or pictures of Gods at their bedside and these items need to be treated with great care and respect.

Dying and death

Death in hospital can cause considerable religious distress to a Hindu patient and their family. Therefore, many patients may have a strong desire, and should be allowed, to die at home. If in hospital they will need to be surrounded by their family who may wish to read passages from holy texts, say prayers with and for them, and perform required ceremonies.

After death real distress may be caused if a non-Hindu touches the body without wearing disposable gloves. Unless otherwise advised by the family, close the eyes and straighten the legs. Do not cut the hair, nails or beard. Hands should be placed on the chest with the palms together and fingers under the chin. Religious objects or jewellery should not be removed. Wrap the body in a plain white sheet.

Judaism

Jews consider themselves to be a nation as much as a religious community. The religious aspects of Judaism are based on the relationship between God and man, and relationships between individual humans based on principles of fairness and equality. Religious observance is a means of publicly displaying a personal acceptance of a close connection between the individual and God. Orthodox Jews are very devout in their faith and adhere strictly to the ancient Torah (holy scriptures/laws). Reform or Liberal Jews believe in the Torah but interpret the laws and scriptures in relation to modern-day circumstances.

Considerations for practice

Personal hygiene

Orthodox Jews may wish to wash themselves before and after eating. Running water is required for this so, if the patient is unable to get out of bed, a bowl and jug of water should be offered.

Diet

Only Kosher food is acceptable to many Jewish patients. Milk and meat are not eaten at the same meal. Meat must be killed according to Kosher ritual and is acceptable only from animals that chew the cud and have cloven hooves, or poultry. Pig and rabbit are forbidden. Fish must have fins and scales and therefore shellfish are forbidden. If Kosher meals are not available, a vegetarian diet should be offered.

Prayer

Jews usually say prayers three times a day and privacy and peace should be given to allow this to happen. The Sabbath is a holy day on which Jews are restricted in what they may do. It begins at sunset on Friday and ends at sunset on Saturday. It is important to establish the patient's principles with regard to the Sabbath as they may significantly impact on the care offered during this time (for example, a patient may not be willing to use a pen to sign their name on forms).

Death and dying

A Jew who is dying may wish to hear or recite special psalms (particularly Psalm 23). After death the body should be touched by care staff as little as possible and disposable gloves should be worn at all times. Contact should be made with either the next of kin or the rabbi as soon as possible as they will arrange for the preparation of the body. The face should be covered with a clean cloth or sheet, arms should not be crossed but left at the side of the body with palms facing inwards. Any catheters, drains and tubes should be left in place, as should any wound dressings. Open wounds should be covered. If the patient dies at night the light should be left on when there is no one in the room or bed space. Female bodies should be attended to by female care staff and, if at all possible, male bodies by male care staff.

Islam

Islam means 'submission and peace' and includes acceptance of those articles of faith, commands and ordinances revealed through the prophet Mohammed. Muslims follow the Islamic faith and believe that the whole universe is under the direction of Allah and nothing can happen unless he wills it. Most practising Muslims follow five main duties or pillars of Islam:

- faith in one God;
- prayer at five set times every day;
- give a required amount to charity each year;
- fast during the holy month of Ramadan;
- make a pilgrimage (Hajj) once in their lives to Mecca if they can.

Considerations for practice

Physical examination/procedures

Physical examination and procedures should generally be carried out by a member of the health care team who is of the same gender as the patient. Privacy during any procedure is very important and female patients may be reluctant to remove clothing. They may also wish for a family member to act as a chaperone when physical examination/procedures are being carried out. Consideration should be given to ensure that the patient remains covered appropriately throughout the examination and any other procedure that may need to be performed as part of the care provided. Care must be taken not to remove any jewellery without the patient's/family's permission as it often has a special or religious significance to the patient.

Personal hygiene

In general Muslims prefer to wash in running water so a shower is preferable to a bath where possible.

Diet

Meat must be slaughtered according to the Halal ritual in which the meat is drained of blood. Halal beef, lamb and chicken are eaten but pork, carrion and blood are forbidden. Fish and eggs are allowed but must not be cooked where pork and other non-Halal meat is cooked (for example in a hospital or care home kitchen). During the month of Ramadan a Muslim must fast between sunrise and sunset. Although Muslims who are temporarily ill or who have a chronic condition may be permitted not to fast, it is important for health care staff to understand that the fasting may still compromise medical diets, tests, etc. If Halal food is not available the family should be allowed to bring food in for the patient, or a strict vegetarian diet should be offered.

Medication

Islam prohibits the consumption of alcohol so therefore they may refuse medication that contains alcohol.

Prayer

Devout Muslims will pray up to five times a day. Privacy and peace should be given to allow them to do this. Before prayer a ritual wash in running water is undertaken in which face, hands and arms are washed in a predetermined way. If the patient is confined to bed they may need help with their preparation for prayer and a jug of water and a bowl will ensure a source of running water is available. Clothes should also be changed if they have become soiled. There is a special format for prayer that uses special hand gestures instead of whole body movements that can be carried out when the patient is confined to bed.

Family and the individual

Muslim patients tend to be visited frequently by their extended family, which can cause some difficulties with regard to the preset visiting times and 'numbers of visitor' policies that exist in most UK hospitals. Many of the visitors may also wish to be involved in the care of the patient, so they should be advised on how they may contribute. As Muslims do not generally encourage men and women to mix freely in public, Muslim patients should not be placed in mixed wards.

Death and dying

As the person approaches death they will expect to have their family and friends around them, which sometimes can mean a considerable number of people visiting at any one time. If this happens, caring for the patient in a side room may be preferable. If members of the family are not in attendance when death occurs, health care staff should wear disposable gloves so that they do not directly touch the body. The person's head should be turned towards Mecca (usually southeast in the UK), the arms and legs straightened, eyes and mouth closed and the body covered entirely with a clean white sheet. Female bodies should be attended to by female care staff and, if at all possible, male bodies by male care staff. The remaining preparation of the body will be carried out by a member of the family, who should be contacted immediately.

Sikhism

'Sikh' translates roughly as 'student or disciple' and originated as a reformist movement of Hinduism; its founder, Guru Nanak, attempting to combine the best features of Hinduism and Islam. Sikhs believe in one God and they must live a spiritual life and develop their own individual relationship with God by dedicating their lives to doing good. Thus, while on this earth they should be truthful, gentle, kind and generous, and work towards the common good. They perceive all men as equal.

Sikhs have five 'signs', which they should wear at all times, known as the 'five Ks'. They are:

> Kesh – uncut beard and hair;
> Kangha – wooden comb;
> Kara – a steel bracelet worn on the right wrist;
> Kirpan – a sharp knife with a double-edged blade (often now in the
> UK worn in the form of a badge/brooch);
> Kaccha – long underpants/trousers.

Considerations for practice

Physical examination

Generally, Sikh men and women would prefer to be examined by a member of the health care staff of the same gender as themselves, and would wish to remain as covered as possible through an examination or procedure. Removal of any of the five Ks must be strictly with the agreement/permission of the patient or their family. When removed they should be treated with great care.

Personal hygiene

Sikhs prefer to use running water for washing and thus prefer to shower rather than bathe. If a patient is unable to use a shower, a bowl and a jug of water is an acceptable alternative. Male Sikhs may also need help to remove their turban (which has to be done at least once a day). Both men and women may need help with the required regular washing, drying and combing of their hair.

Diet

Meat that has been prepared in a ritualistic way for another religion should not be given to a Sikh. Although there are no specific rules about not eating meat, many Sikhs are vegetarian and this includes not eating fish or eggs.

Prayer

Sikhs spend a lot of time in meditative contemplation of God. Before prayers the person will want to wash themselves and dress in clean clothes if necessary. A patient may need help to ensure this happens.

Family and the individual

Visiting the sick is a duty in the Sikh community, so the patient may receive many visitors. Families and friends will also expect to be involved in discussions about treatment and the provision of health care. A patient may refuse treatment or care if the family does not agree with it. Men or women should not be placed in mixed wards.

Death and dying

If a member of the family is not available, health care staff should wear disposable gloves to avoid direct contact with the patient after death. Do not undress, wash the body or remove any of the five Ks as that is something the family would wish to carry out themselves. Drains and other tubes can be removed. The body should then be wrapped in a clean white cloth/sheet ready for the family to care for.

Buddhism

Buddhism is a way of life rather than an organised religion. Its focus is on personal spiritual development and the attainment of a deeper insight into the true nature of life, rather than on a set of ritualistic practices. It teaches that all life is interconnected and the path to enlightenment is through the practice and development of morality, meditation and wisdom. The practice of Buddhism is extremely diverse and Buddhists from different regions will have different interpretations of the central ideas.

Considerations for practice

Diet

Most Buddhists are vegetarians.

Medication

Some Buddhists may refuse to accept medication that contains alcohol or animal products. Some may prefer to use alternative strategies, such as meditation, to relieve pain as an option to conventional analgesia.

Dying

A Buddhist who knows that they are dying will probably wish to have their family and friends with them to meditate and chant mantras as death approaches. They will need as much peace and quiet as possible to allow this to happen. After death, do not touch or move the body of a Buddhist patient until advice has been sought from an appropriate source (for example, the family, friends or the hospital chaplain).

(Clarke,1993; Weller, 1997; Henley and Schott,1999)

www.ethnicityonline.net

SUMMARY

Working with cultural diversity requires knowledge and sensitivity. Generally, patients and family members would prefer to be asked about their customs and religious requirements rather than just ignoring them. The most important thing to remember is that whatever cultural or religious beliefs a patient may hold, they will still have preferences and needs that are individual and personal to them alone.

Further reading

Further information on a range of religions and implications for practice in respect of health care can be obtained from the internet. Your starting point could include: **www.interfaith.org.uk**; **www.bbc.co.uk/religion/religions.**

LEGISLATION AND POLICY

As a nurse there are two main pieces of legislation relating to cultural diversity that you need to be familiar with.

The Human Rights Act 1998

The Human Rights Act came into force in October 2000. It represents the translation of the law of the European Convention on Human Rights into British law. This has meant that, for the first time, Britain has a legislative framework that defines standards for what each person has a right to expect with regard to fundamental human rights and freedoms. The Act covers all infringements of human rights regardless of gender, disability, ethnic identity, sexuality or class and makes it unlawful for public authorities (which includes NHS Trusts, Primary Care Trusts, all health authorities, private and voluntary-sector contractors, social services, General Practitioners, dentists, opticians and pharmacists) to act in a way that is incompatible with Convention rights, unless they are acting under legislation which makes it impossible to act differently. The Convention rights include the following.

- **Article 2: The right to life** – The state is required to make adequate provision in its laws for the protection of human life. This means it must take positive steps to protect life in all kinds of situations including admission to hospital/health care. Hospitals are under a duty to take positive steps to safeguard a patient's right to life. Relevant health care staff may therefore need to consider the implications before refusing life-saving treatment to a patient.
- **Article 3: Freedom from torture and inhuman or degrading treatment or punishment** – An absolute right not to be tortured or subjected to treatment or punishment that is inhuman or degrading. How an individual's treatment is classified depends on many different factors including their state of health. Whether or not treatment is considered degrading depends on 'whether a reasonable person of the same age or sex and health as you would have felt degraded' (Department for Constitutional Affairs, 2006, p.16).
- **Article 4: Freedom from slavery and forced or compulsory labour** – An absolute right not be treated like a slave or forced to perform certain kinds of labour. This might apply to a situation such as staff from overseas having their passports removed by their employers to prevent them leaving a place of work.
- **Article 5: Right to liberty, freedom and security of person** – Unless a detention is lawful, an individual cannot be deprived of their liberty for even a short period of time. Detention in this context can include

within mental hospitals. Acceptable reasons for arrest and detention, in accordance with set procedures set down by law, include: if a person is shown to be of unsound mind, an alcoholic, a drug addict or a vagrant, or to prevent an individual spreading infectious disease.

- **Article 6: Right to a fair trial** – Every person has the right to a fair hearing, a public hearing, an independent and impartial tribunal and a hearing within a reasonable time.
- **Article 7: Freedom from retrospective criminal law and no punishment without law** – This relates to the right to normally not be found guilty of a criminal offence that occurred at a time when the person was not aware that it was a criminal act.
- **Article 8: Right to respect for private and family life, home and correspondence** – This confers the right for each person to live their own life as is reasonable within a democratic society and takes account of the freedoms and rights of others. This right can also include the right to have information about the person like, for example, official records including medical information, kept private and confidential. This right also places restrictions on the extent to which any public authority can invade an individual's privacy about their body without their permission. It should be noted that this raises issues in such procedures as taking blood samples and the right to refuse treatment.
- **Article 9: Freedom of thought, conscience and religion** – This provides an absolute right for a person to hold the thoughts, positions of conscience or religion of their choice. This includes the right for the person to practise or demonstrate their religion in private or public (as long as it does not interfere with the rights and freedoms of others).
- **Article 10: Freedom of expression** – 'Expression' here includes personal views or opinions, speaking aloud, publication of articles or books or leaflets, television or radio broadcasting, producing works of art, communication through the internet, some forms of commercial information (DCA, 2006, p.23).
- **Article 11: Freedom of assembly and association** – Every person has the right to 'peacefully' assemble with others.
- **Article 12: Right to marry** – This includes the right to have a family.
- **Article 14: Freedom from discrimination** – In the context of the Act, discrimination is defined as 'treating people in similar situations differently, or those in different situations in the same way, without proper justification' (DCA, 2006, p. 25). Among other issues this includes associated sex and sexual orientation, age, race, colour, language, religion, disability, political or other opinion, national or social origin, association with a national minority, property, birth (for example whether born inside or outside of marriage), and marital

status. Regardless of status, everyone is entitled to equal access to all the rights set out in the Act.

- **Protocol 1 of Article 2: Right to education** – No person should be denied the right to the education system and an effective education.

Articles 2, 3, 8, 9 and 14 are particularly important to nursing practice and relate to the Nursing and Midwifery Council's *Code* (2008).

Activity

Access further information regarding the Human Rights Act 1998 from **www.direct.gov.uk**, **www.YourRights.org.uk**, **www.dh.gov.uk** or through a general search engine such as Google. Then consider and note down the implications of Articles 2, 3, 8, 9 and 14 in relation to your practice as a student of nursing.

The Race Relations (Amendment) Act 2000

The Race Relations (Amendment) Act 2000 strengthened the 1976 Race Relations Act and includes the requirement that all scheduled public authorities must have due regard to the need:

- to eliminate unlawful discrimination;
- to promote equality of opportunity and good relations between persons of different racial backgrounds.

These duties cover all aspects of an organisation's activities, policy and service delivery/provision as well as employment practices. This obviously has considerable implications for your work as a nurse, both as a student and a qualified practitioner.

Further reading

Further reading regarding the Race Relations (Amendment) Act 2000 can be obtained from **www.homeoffice.gov.uk**

REFERENCES

Andrews, M.M. and Boyle, J.S. (2007) *Transcultural Concepts in Nursing Care* (5th edn). London: Lippincott Williams and Wilkins

Clarke, P.B. (1993) *The World's Religions*. London: Readers Digest

Commission for Racial Equality (2007) *Race, Ethnicity and National Origin*. Available at **http://83.137.212.42/sitearchive/cre/diversity/wordsandmeanings/essay2.html** (accessed 7/12/2008)

Department for Constitutional Affairs (2006) *A Guide to the Human Rights Act 1998* (3rd edn). London: DCA

Geiger, J. and Davidhizar, R. (2007) *Transcultural Nursing: Assessment and intervention* (5th edn). New York: Mosby

Henley, A. and Schott, J. (1999) *Culture, Religion and Patient Care in a Multi-Ethnic Society: A handbook for professionals*. London: Age Concern

Hofstede, G. and Hofstede, G.J. (2004) *Cultures and Organisations: Software of the mind* (2nd edn). New York: McGraw-Hill

Human Rights Act (1998) Available at **www.direct.gov.uk** (accessed 7/12/08)

Jirwe, M. (2008) *Cultural Competence in Nursing*. Stockholm: Karolinska Institute

Leininger, M. and McFarland, M. (2002) *Transcultural Nursing* (3rd edn). New York: McGraw-Hill

Macionis, J.J. and Plummer, K. (2005) *Sociology: A global introduction* (3rd edn). Harlow: Pearson Education

Nursing and Midwifery Council (2008) *Standards of conduct, performance and ethics for nurses and midwives*. London: NMC

Office of Population Census and Surveys (2001). Available at: **www.gov.uk** (accessed 7/12/08)

Papadopoulos, I. (ed.) (2006) *Transcultural Health and Social Care: Development of culturally competent practitioners*. Oxford: Elsevier

Race Relations (Amendment) Act 2000. Available at **www.homeoffice.gov.uk** (accessed 7/12/08)

Royal College of Nursing (2006) *Transcultural Health Care Practice: An educational resource for nurses and health care practitioners*. Available at **www.rcn.org.uk/resources/transcultural/index.php** (accessed 7/12/08).

Wagner, A.L. (2002) 'Nursing students' development of caring through creative reflective practice', cited in Freshwater, D. (ed.) *Therapeutic Nursing: Improving patient care through self-awareness and reflection*. London: Sage

Weller, P. (ed.) (1997) *Religions in the UK: A multi-faith directory.* Derby: University of Derby

Useful websites

www.ethnicityonline.net (accessed 7/12/08)

Chapter 7

Quality Assurance

The aim of this chapter is to introduce the quality assurance framework guiding health care provision in the United Kingdom and, in particular, in England. Quality assurance is obviously expected wherever you work, but what tends to be different is both the context and the framework that monitor and guide the assurance around the quality.

Outcomes

On completion of this chapter you should be able to:

- understand some of the main policies and procedures that inform and guide quality assurance in the provision of health care;

- briefly outline the concept of clinical governance and clinical audit;

- understand issues relevant to risk assessment and vulnerable adults;

- understand the importance of patients' and users' views in quality assurance;

- briefly outline the key steps in the development of Integrated Care Pathways.

DEFINING QUALITY ASSURANCE

According to Marr and Giebing (1994, p.18), at its simplest, 'quality assurance is about describing, measuring and taking action'. Within the context of health care, Ball (1989, cited in Clarke and Copcutt, 1997, p. 211) defines quality assurance as 'taking positive action to assess and evaluate performance against agreed and defined standards in order to create and manage a service which regularly achieves desired levels of care and service'. Irwin and Fordham (1995, p. 10) suggest that for health care professionals it is 'essentially about practitioners being systematic as well as intuitive in evaluating the care they provide and continually seeking to improve it'.

Quality assurance associated with the provision and delivery of health care is, in fact, relatively new. Prior to the 1980s quality assurance within the health service tended to be implicit rather than explicit, owing largely, according to Dowding and Barr (2002), to the fact that health care was felt to exist for altruistic motives rather than for profit, and these motives were not open to quality scrutiny. International influences in 1984 led to the British government launching the National Quality Campaign for both public and private industries, and within this the NHS was strongly encouraged to ensure quality control systems were in place. By the 1990s specific requirements and advice on quality were being set out in government health policy. For example, The Patients' Charter (Department of Health, 1991) set down precise national standards regarding various rights and expectations for all patients. Subsequent policy and legislation, including *A First Class Service: Improving quality in the new NHS* (Department of Health, 1998), made more specific plans for progress in improving the health service, especially in terms of effectiveness, efficiency and excellence. These plans reflected the need for clear lines of responsibility and quality-management activities incorporating monitoring and continuous improvement. *A First Class Service* also identified clinical effectiveness, evidence-based practice, clinical supervision and continuing professional development activities as specific requirements for health care practitioners in support of quality assurance.

THE ORGANISATION OF QUALITY ASSURANCE IN UK HEALTH CARE

Sale (2005) suggests that within the health service the main levels at which quality processes take place are:

- at national level;
- at Strategic Health Authority/NHS Trust level;
- at the local clinical level.

National level

There is no easy way to introduce you to the plethora of organisations and agencies with a mandate to ensure quality of care provision at national level. However, you need to have a basic understanding/awareness of the key agencies as you will encounter their work either directly or indirectly in your practice.

Care Quality Commission

The Care Quality Commission is the independent regulator of health and social care in England. It regulates health and adult social care services, whether provided by the NHS, local authorities, private companies or voluntary organisations. It is also responsible for protecting the rights of people detained under the Mental Health Act.

The Commission's role is to ensure that essential common quality standards are being met where care is provided and work towards the improvement of these care services. The Commission promotes the rights and interests of people who use services and it has a wide range of enforcement powers to take action on people's behalf if services are unacceptably poor. Its main activities include:

- the registration of health and social care providers to ensure they are meeting essential common quality standards;
- monitoring and inspection of all health and adult social care;
- using enforcement powers, such as fines and public warnings or closures, if standards are not being met;
- improving health and social care services by undertaking regular reviews of how well those who arrange and provide services locally are performing;
- providing special reviews on particular care services, pathways of care or themes where there are particular concerns about quality;
- reporting the outcomes of their work so that people who use services have information about the quality of their local health and adult social care services.

It regulates health and social care activities such as:

- personal care;
- accommodation for people who require nursing or personal care;
- accommodation for people who require treatment for drug and alcohol misuse;
- accommodation and nursing or personal care in the further education sector;
- surgical procedures;
- diagnostic procedures;
- treatment of disease, disorder or injury;

- services in slimming clinics;
- transport services, triage and medical advice provided remotely;
- maternity and midwifery services;
- termination of pregnancy;
- assessment of medical treatment for persons detained under the Mental Health Act 1983;
- nursing care;
- management and supply of blood and blood-derived products.

Another important part of its work is collecting data from service users' experiences of care services. In some cases it involves patients and their carers directly in working alongside its inspectors to give an expert user view of services.

It makes use of all informal and formal information and data to monitor what is happening inside health and social care systems as well as across both health and social care in order to identify where a pattern of incidents indicates that something untoward may be happening.

The Care Quality Commission does not have a remit in Scotland or Northern Ireland.

www.cqc.org.uk

National Patient Safety Agency (NPSA)

The NPSA is an 'arm's-length' body of the Department of Health set up to lead and contribute to improved, safe patient care by informing, supporting and influencing organisations and people working in the UK health care sector. There are three divisions of the NPSA.

- **National Reporting and Learning Service (NRLS)** – its aim is to help improve patient care in the NHS with rapid response to incidents, analysis of incidents that come via the National Reporting and Learning system and by taking the lead on national initiatives to improve patient safety.

www.npsa.nhs.uk

- **National Clinical Assessment Service (NCAS)** – works with health organisations and individual practitioners where there is concern about the performance of a dentist, doctor or pharmacist. The NCAS covers the UK and both the NHS and independent sectors of health care.

www.ncas.nspa.nhs.uk

- **National Research Ethics Service (NRES)** – seeks to protect the rights, safety, dignity and well-being of research participants who are part of clinical trials and other research within the NHS.

  www.nres.npsa.nhs.uk

NHS complaints procedure

This complaints procedure covers complaints made by a patient or person about any matter connected with the provision of NHS services by NHS organisations or primary care practitioners (GPs, dentists, opticians and pharmacists). The procedure also covers services provided overseas or by the private sector where the NHS has paid for them. If an individual is dissatisfied with the treatment or service they have received from the NHS, they are entitled to make a complaint, have it considered, and receive a response from the NHS organisation or primary care practitioner concerned (except for Foundation Trusts, which must have in place their own systems for the internal handling of complaints at local resolution level, which may differ from that outlined above. However, the independent review stage is still carried out by the Care Quality Commission). The complaint can also be made by someone acting on behalf of the patient or person with their consent. The complaint must normally be made within six months of the event(s) or within six months of becoming aware that the person has something to complain about.

The first stage of the procedure is known as 'local resolution', with the complaint, in the first instance, being made to the organisation or primary care practitioner who provided the services. Initially this may be by voicing concerns to a member of staff or the Patient Advice and Liaison Service (PALS). However, if the individual wishes to make the complaint more formal they can do so either orally or in writing (including e.mail) to a complaints manager. A reply from a primary care practitioner involved should be expected within 10 working days, and from a NHS organisation within 25 working days. If the individual is not satisfied with the outcome they can request/agree an 'independent review'. In England such reviews are carried out by the Care Quality Commission. If the person is still dissatisfied it is possible for the complaint to be considered by a completely independent Health Service Ombudsman (investigator of complaints). Financial compensation, legal action and professional misconduct are not dealt with through this process.

www.dh.gov.uk

Further reading

Further information on monitoring and promoting improvement of quality of health care in Wales, Scotland and Northern Ireland can be obtained from: **www.hiw.org.uk**, **www.nhshealthquality.org.uk** and **www.dhsspsni.gov.uk**

The Health and Social Care Act 2008 includes measures which seek to ensure the provision and delivery of safe and high-quality services. Details can be obtained from **www.dh.gov. uk/en/Publicationsandstatistics/Legislation/Actsandbills/ HealthandSocialCareBill/index.htm** For current information regarding the complaints procedures go to **www.dh.gov.uk** and type 'complaints procedure' into the search box.

Strategic Health Authority, NHS Trust/PCT level

These organisations are responsible for ensuring that the quality of provision of service is in accordance with requirements set at national level. One mechanism they must have in place, through which they can demonstrate this responsibility at this level, is a clinical governance framework.

Clinical governance

Clinical governance is a very broad concept. Introduced in 1998, it located quality at the centre of proposed NHS reforms by building on earlier efforts to audit, monitor and improve practice. The Department of Health defined it as:

> a framework through which organizations are accountable for continuously improving the quality of their services and safeguarding high standards of care by creating an environment in which excellence in clinical care will flourish.
>
> (Department of Health, 1998, p. 33)

The Royal College of Nursing identifies clinical governance as 'a framework which helps all clinicians – including nurses – to continuously improve quality and safeguard standards of care' (RCN, 1998, cited in RCN, 2003, p. 7). Som (2004) sought to encompass the complexity of the contributing factors and organisation-wide implications for continuous quality improvement, stating that:

> Clinical governance is defined as a governance system for healthcare organisations that promotes an integrated approach towards management of inputs, structures and processes to improve the outcome of health-care service delivery where health staff work in an environment of greater accountability for clinical quality.
>
> (Som, 2004, p. 89)

Covering the organisation's systems and processes for monitoring and improving services, the key elements of clinical governance include:

- strong leadership and accountability;
- patient, public, carer consultation and involvement;
- clinical effectiveness and commitment to quality;
- education, training and continuous professional development;
- research and development;
- clinical risk management;
- staff management and performance;
- use of information about patients' experiences, outcomes and processes.

(All of the key elements are of equal value and importance and all are interrelated.)

In essence clinical governance is perceived as being about ensuring safe, high-quality care from those involved in a patient's journey, while ensuring the patient remains the main focus and priority. Baggott (2004) identifies clinical governance at Trust level as including the following processes.

- **Clear lines of responsibility and accountability for clinical areas.** NHS Trusts (and PCTs) have a duty of quality whereby the chief executive is responsible for the quality of services provided, and each Trust has a named senior officer whose responsibility it is to ensure that arrangements for clinical governance are effective.
- **A comprehensive programme of quality improvement**. This includes involvement in clinical audit and confidential enquiries, a commitment to evidence-based practice, and to the implementation of clinical standards in National Service Frameworks (NSF) and National Institute for Health and Clinical Excellence (NICE) recommendations. There is

also a responsibility to ensure that workforce planning and continuing professional development are consistent with the need to constantly improve services. Trusts and PCTs are also required to demonstrate that effective communication systems, both internally and externally, and efficient information management processes, are in place.

- **Procedures for identifying and remedying poor performance.** This includes complaints procedures, incident reporting and clear policies for reporting of concerns of staff.
- **Clear policies for identifying and minimising risk**. Trusts and PCTs must have clear policies in place for identifying and minimising risk.

Minimising risk – risk assessment

O'Rourke (2005) suggests risk assessment in its simplest form is a process that seeks to identify, evaluate and address potential and actual risks. The increased awareness in recent years that risk assessment and the management of risk, within the health and social care sectors, are important factors in providing a high-quality service can, according to Milligan (2003), be linked to the professional and government initiative to modernise and monitor health care provision.

With a commitment to improve risk assessment, a report commissioned by the government in 2000, *An Organization With a Memory: Report of an expert group on learning from adverse events in the NHS*, was published (Department of Health, 2000a). The remit of the group was to:

- review what was then known regarding the scale and nature of serious failures within health care;
- examine the extent to which the NHS had the capacity to learn from such failures;
- recommend measures that minimised possibilities of them happening again.

After accepting the recommendations of the report, the government published *Building a Safer NHS for Patients: Implementing an organization with a memory* (Department of Health, 2001a). This document identified government plans for promoting patient safety and established it as part of their drive for quality within the NHS. Since then a number of reports, for example *Safety First – A report for patients, clinicians and health care managers* (2006a), have been published, all with recommendations that seek to continue to improve patient safety.

Further reading

Further information on clinical governance can be accessed at:
**www.dh.gov.uk/en/Publicationsandstatistics/Lettersandcirculars/
Healthservicecirculars/DH_4004883**
This website provides succinct but relatively comprehensive
coverage of the government's aims and policy principles and
information on the implementation of clinical governance in the
NHS.
**www.rcn.org.uk/publications/pdf/ClinicalGovernance2003.
pdf** This Royal College of Nursing guide summarises the key
themes of clinical governance and includes case studies to show its
application.

Further reading in support of the wider concept/context of risk
assessment can also include:
Health and Safety Executive
The Health and Safety Commission is responsible for health
and safety regulation in Great Britain. The Health and Safety
Executive and local government are the enforcing authorities who
work in support of the Commission. Further information can be
obtained from **www.hse.gov.uk**.

Medicines and Healthcare Products Regulatory Agency
Its role is to 'enhance and safeguard the health of the public
by ensuring that medicines and medical devices work, and are
acceptably safe'. Further information can be obtained from
www.mhra.gov.uk.

Information regarding risk assessment (health care) in Wales can
be obtained from **www.hiw.org.uk**, in Scotland from
www.nhshealthquality.org, and in Northern Ireland from
www.northernireland.gov.uk.

Whistle-blowing case studies are available from:
www.nhsemployers.org/practice/whistleblowing.cfm These
provide a useful opportunity to examine some situations on
reporting and addressing concerns relevant to the provision of
health care.

Local clinical level

Quality assurance at local level covers a variety of activities including clinical audit, patients' and users' views and patient advisory services. Further issues such as Protection of Vulnerable Adults, Integrated Care Pathways and the *Essence of Care* (Department of Health, 2001b) initiative can also be included here.

Clinical audit

Clinical audit is a quality improvement process that was introduced by the 1989 White Paper *Working for Patients*. The Department of Health in 1989 defined clinical audit as:

> . . . the systematic and critical analysis of the quality of clinical care, including the procedures used for diagnosis, treatment and care, the associated use of resources and the resulting outcome and quality of life for the patient.
>
> (Department of Health, 1989)

Currently, NICE describes it as:

> a quality improvement process that seeks to improve the patient care and outcomes through systematic review of the care against explicit criteria and implementation of change.
>
> **www.nice.org.uk**

Essentially then, clinical audit is about clinical effectiveness and quality improvement. It is now a key component of the clinical governance framework and is well established both within the NHS and the independent sector. The key elements of clinical audit are:

- setting standards/criteria for a chosen area/topic;
- measuring current practice;
- comparing the results with the standards/criteria set;
- changing practice if required;
- re-auditing to ensure quality practice has been maintained or practice has improved.

Put together, these elements are usually referred to as the 'audit cycle'.

The fundamental principles associated with clinical audit are that it:

- should be professionally led;
- should be viewed as an educational process;

- should be a routine part of clinical practice;
- should be based on the setting of standards;
- generates results based on the setting of standards;
- generates results that can be used to improve the outcome of quality care;
- involves management in both the process and outcome of audit;
- should be confidential at the individual patient/clinician level;
- should be informed by the views of patients/clients.

(NHS Executive, 1994)

Further reading

Further information on clinical audit can be obtained from: **www.rcn.org.uk** (type 'quality improvement – clinical audit' into search box). This website provides a range of information relevant to clinical audit.
www.nice.org.uk/usingguidance/implementationtools/auditadvice and follow the pdf link. This website provides comprehensive coverage of principles for best practice in clinical audit.

Patients' and users' views

Over the past decade there has been a clear move by the government towards a culture of regularly involving and consulting patients and the public in decision-making and service improvement. In 2003 the Health and Social Care Act set out legislation that placed a duty on the NHS to engage actively with community and service users. In October 2008 this was taken a stage further when the government published the Local Government and Public Health Act (2008). This Act contained new duties for health organisations to reinforce and improve the way the NHS pays attention to and utilises the views of the public to improve local health services. As part of this process the Act introduced the establishment of Local Involvement Networks (LINKs).

Local Involvement Networks (LINKs)

From October 2008 a network of local individuals, groups and organisations was set up to cover all publicly funded health and social care services. The Act sets out LINKs activities as:

- promoting and supporting the involvement of people in commissioning, provision and scrutiny of local care services;

- enabling people to monitor, and review, the commissioning and provision of local services;
- obtaining the views of people about their needs for, and their experiences of local care services;
- making the views of local people known, and reporting and making recommendations about how local care services might be improved, to persons responsible for commissioning, providing, managing or scrutinising local care services.

The specific NHS duties relating to LINKs include the following:

- NHS providers are under a duty to allow LINKs to enter and view certain health and social care facilities.
- PCTs are under a duty to respond within a particular timescale to all reports and recommendations made by LINKs.
- All NHS bodies are required, under the Freedom of Information Act, to provide information within a particular timescale.
                         www.library.nhs.uk/healthmanagement

The NHS Centre for Involvement (NCI) has been appointed by the government to support and act as the lead organisation for LINKs.

NHS National Patient Survey Programme

The National Patient Survey Programme, co-ordinated by the Care Quality Commission, gathers feedback from patients on different aspects of the experience of care they have recently received, across a variety of services/settings. These care experiences include inpatients, outpatients, emergency care, maternity care, mental health services, primary care services and ambulance services. The results are used:

- by PCTs and SHAs to track their performance over time and inform improvement activities;
- by the Care Quality Commission as performance indicators to feed into their annual health check for all NHS organisations;
- by the Department of Health to measure progress against Public Service Agreements.
                                               www.dh.gov.uk

The Patient Advisory Liaison Service (PALS)

Established in every NHS and Primary Care Trust this service has been set up to offer confidential support and advice directly to service users, families and carers if they have a perceived cause for complaint or concern. Although not part of the complaints procedure itself, they liaise with staff, managers and, where appropriate, other relevant organisations, to informally negotiate and encourage fast solution of the problem or concern. The core functions of PALS are to:

- be identifiable and accessible to patients, their carers, friends and families;
- provide on-the-spot help in every Trust with the power to negotiate immediate solutions or speedy resolution of problems;
- act as a gateway to appropriate independent advice and advocacy support from local and national sources;
- provide accurate information to patients, carers and families, about the Trust's services, and about other health-related issues;
- act as a catalyst for change and improvement by providing the Trust with information and feedback on problems arising and gaps in services;
- operate within a local network with other PALS in their area and work across organisational boundaries;
- support staff at all levels within the Trust to develop a responsive culture.

www.pals.nhs.uk

Further issues

Protection of vulnerable adults

Risk assessment in health and social care also involves the protection of vulnerable adults. A vulnerable adult is defined broadly as:

> a person who is or may be in need of community care services by reason of mental or other disabilities, age or illness; and who is or may be unable to take care of him or herself, or unable to protect him or herself against significant harm or exploitation.
>
> (Department of Health, 2000b)

Following a number of high-profile and serious incidents involving vulnerable adults the Department of Health published the *No Secrets: Guidance on developing and implementing multi-agency policies and procedures to protect vulnerable adults from abuse* (2000b) document. This document provides guidance on actions to be taken within health and social care regarding the appropriate protection and support of vulnerable adults. The aim of the guidance has been to construct a framework in which all relevant agencies are required to work together to ensure that strong and coherent policies and procedures are in place, and implemented locally, for the protection of vulnerable adults who are at risk of abuse. Abuse in this context is defined by the Department of Health (2000b,

p. 9) as 'a violation of an individual's human and civil rights by another person or persons'. The abuse may be a single or repeated act, occur in any relationship and may result in serious harm to, or exploitation of, the person subject to it. The main forms of abuse can be identified as:

- **physical abuse** (includes misuse of medication and restraint);
- **sexual abuse;**
- **psychological abuse** (includes verbal abuse, controlling and withdrawal from services or supportive networks);
- **financial/material abuse** (includes theft, fraud and misuse or misappropriation of possessions);
- **neglect and acts of omission** (includes ignoring medical or physical care needs and withholding necessities of life such as medication and adequate nutrition);
- **discriminatory abuse** (includes racist, sexist and ageist abuse and harassment).

A further form of abuse referring specifically to neglect and poor professional practice is often referred to as 'institutional abuse'. This may be an isolated event of poor or unsatisfactory professional practice through to ongoing ill treatment, or gross misconduct.

The NMC defines abuse within the registrant–client relationship as 'the result of the misuse of power or a betrayal of trust, respect or intimacy between the registrant and the client, which the registrant should know would cause physical or emotional harm to the client' (NMC, 2009, p. 2). Its guidance, which defines the standards of conduct within the registrant/client/patient relationship, identifies zero tolerance of abuse as the only philosophy consistent with protecting the public. It stresses that registrants have a responsibility for ensuring they safeguard the interests of their clients at all times and to protect patients/clients from all forms of abuse. If, in the course of their professional practice, registrants suspect or believe that a client is being or has been abused, they must report this as soon as practical to a person of appropriate authority. This zero tolerance of abuse is also expected from students of nursing.

Activity

It is recommended that you access and read a copy of the guidelines entitled *Registrant/client relationships and prevention of abuse* from **www.nmc-org.uk**

The Care Standards Act (Department of Health, 2000c) outlined a requirement for the introduction of a Protection of Vulnerable Adults (POVA) register. This register was set up in England and Wales in 2004 and, managed by the Department of Health, contains a list of people deemed unsuitable to work with vulnerable adults. People are referred to and included on the list if they have abused or harmed vulnerable adults in their care or placed them at risk of harm (whether or not in the course of their employment). Any persons placed on the register may not be employed in any capacity to work with vulnerable adults. Checks are made when an individual applies for a position with a new employer, moves or is transferred from a non-care position to a position working with vulnerable adults. This scheme currently applies to registered service providers in care homes, domiciliary agencies and adult placement schemes, and all persons working with vulnerable adults in either a paid or a voluntary capacity must be checked against the register. Employment agencies and businesses who supply care workers to these providers are also included.

These arrangements will stay in place until a new vetting and barring system identified in The Safeguarding of Vulnerable Groups Act (Department of Health, 2006b) is implemented at some time in 2009. The government's intention is to eventually extend the scheme into the NHS, independent hospitals, clinics and other facilities.

Further reading

Further information related to the *No Secrets: Guidance on developing and implementing multi-agency policies and procedures to protect vulnerable adults from abuse* (2000b) document and the protection of vulnerable adults can be accessed from **www.dh.gov.uk** by following the policy guidance/health and social care links, or from **www.cqc.org.uk**

For current information on the POVA new vetting and barring scheme go to **www.isa-gov.uk** or **www.dh.gov.uk**

For information for Wales go to **www.new.wales.gov.uk**, for Scotland go to **www.scotland.gov.uk** and for Northern Ireland go to **www.nothernireland.gov.uk**

Integrated Care Pathways (ICP)

Integrated Care Pathways may also be known as clinical pathways, multidisciplinary pathways of care, pathways of care, care maps, collaborative care pathways and care profiles. Integrated Care Pathways can be defined as 'structured multidisciplinary care plans which detail essential steps in the care of a patient with a specific clinical problem and describe the expected progress of the patient' (Campbell *et al.*, 1998, p. 133).

The main feature of ICPs is that they are multidisciplinary, locally agreed, evidence-based plans (and records) of care that are patient-focused and that attempt to view the provision of care in terms of the 'patient's journey'. They detail decisions to be made and the care to be provided for a given patient or group for a given condition in a step-wise sequence and within a given timescale. They also incorporate intermediate and long-term outcome criteria and a variance record that allows deviations from the planned care to be documented and analysed. Variations from the pathway may occur as clinical freedom is exercised to meet the needs of the individual patient.

According to Middleton *et al.* (2003), initially the development of such pathways concentrated on specific surgical conditions like, for example, total hip replacement and the more 'predictable' medical conditions such as stroke or acute myocardial infarction, which generally offered a definable sequence of events. However, more and more ICPs are being utilised for less predictable conditions. Because they are locally agreed and developed, it is not possible to provide an overall list of the conditions for which an ICP might have been introduced; however, examples include:

- care of the elderly: acute admission;
- acute pneumonia;
- inflammatory bowel disease;
- asthma;
- prostatectomy;
- mastectomy;
- aortic valve replacement.

A considerable number of benefits are identified in the literature with regard to the use of ICPs and these include:

- encouraging the translation of national guidelines into local protocols and their subsequent application to clinical practice;
- they result in more complete and accessible data collection for audit and encourage changes in practice;

- encouraging multidisciplinary communication and care planning;
- promoting more patient-focused care and improving patient information by letting the patient see what is planned and what progress is expected;
- enabling new staff to learn quickly the key interventions for specific conditions and to appreciate likely variations;
- facilitating multidisciplinary audit and prompt incorporation of improvements in the care into routine practice;
- supporting the introduction of evidence-based practice and use of clinical guidelines;
- they can support continuity and co-ordination of care across different clinical disciplines and sectors;
- providing explicit and well-defined standards for care;
- helping to reduce variations in patient care (by promoting standardisation) and helping to improve clinical outcomes;
- helping to improve and even reduce patient documentation by streamlining and combining multidisciplinary documentation;
- disseminating accepted standards of care;
- providing all carers with information on a client's progress and status;
- making explicit the standards of care against which actual care can be judged;
- patients are able to receive realistic expectations about their conditions and their expected progress;
- full compliance with ICPs meets the NMC standards for clinical record-keeping.

The key steps in developing an ICP are as follows.

- An important area of practice is selected.
- A multidisciplinary team is formed.
- Current clinical evidence for care of the patient group is compared with established clinical guidelines in all areas of practice.
- The ICP is developed (which specifies elements of care detailed in local protocols, the sequence of events and expected patient progress over time).
- The ICP is piloted and the outcomes reviewed.
- If necessary the pathway is revised.
- The ICP is implemented.
- Regular analysis of any variants from the pathway is undertaken (i.e. investigating the reasons why practice was different from that recommended in the ICP).

As a student nurse your involvement in ICPs may include:

- using one in practice;
- developing a pathway for a specific condition;
- evaluating a pathway that has already been developed;
- teaching other members of staff regarding their use.

(Middleton, *et al.* 2003, **www.csp.org.uk**)

Activity

Access further information regarding the development and implementation of ICPs utilising a general search engine such as Google. You should find sample documentation available on many of the sites useful for future practice.

ESSENCE OF CARE

The Department of Health published *The Essence of Care – Patient focused benchmarks for clinical governance* in February 2001. Its aim was to provide a tool that would help practitioners take a patient-focused and structured approach to sharing and comparing practice. It was also designed to support measures to improve quality, and to contribute to clinical governance within organisations. It focuses on what might be described as the fundamental and essential aspects of care and it seeks to enable health care personnel to work with patients to identify best practice and to develop action plans to improve care.

The tool arose from a commitment in *Making a Difference* (Department of Health, 1999), to explore the benefits of benchmarking to help improve quality of care. *The NHS Plan* (Department of Health, 2000d) also reinforces the importance of 'getting the basics right' and of improving the patient experience.

Patients, carers and professionals worked together to agree and describe good-quality care and best practice in 11 areas of care, which are:

- personal and oral hygiene;
- privacy and dignity;

- food and nutrition;
- principles of self-care;
- safety with clients with mental health needs;
- record-keeping;
- pressure ulcers;
- continence and bladder and bowel care;
- communication (between patients, carers and health care personnel);
- promoting health;
- care environment.

(It should be recognised that all sets of benchmarks are interrelated.)

Content of benchmarking toolkit

The *Essence of Care* benchmarking toolkit comprises:

- an overall patient-focused outcome that expresses what patients and/ or carers want from care in a particular area of practice;
- a number of factors that need to be considered in order to achieve the overall patient-focused outcome.

Each factor consists of:

- a patient-focused benchmark of best practice that is placed at the extreme right of the continuum;
- a continuum between poor and best practice – the benchmark for each factor guides users towards best practice;
- indicators for best practice identified by patients, carers and professionals that support the attainment of best practice.

Using clinical benchmarks

Essence of Care benchmarking is a process of comparing, sharing and developing practice in order to achieve and sustain best practice. Changes and improvements focus on the indicators, since these are the items that patients, carers and professionals believed were important in achieving the benchmarks of best practice. The stages involved in benchmarking are highlighted below.

Stage one	Agree best practice.
Stage two	Assess area against best practice.
Stage three	Produce and implement an action plan aimed at achieving best practice.
Stage four	Review achievement towards best practice.
Stage five	Disseminate improvements and/or review the action plan.
Stage six/one	Agree best practice.

The benchmarks are relevant to all health and social care settings. Therefore, the *Essence of Care* is presented in a generic format in order that it can be used in, for example, primary, secondary and tertiary settings and with all patient and/or carer groups, such as in paediatric care, mental health, cancer care, surgery and medicine. It is important that those benchmarking (including patients and carers) agree the indicators that demonstrate best practice within their area of care.

(Department of Health, April 2003)

Activity

It is very important that you understand *Essence of Care* as you will no doubt be involved at some point in its implementation while working as a student of nursing. The full document can be obtained from **www.dh.gov.uk**

REFERENCES

Baggot, R. (2004) *Health and Health Care in Britain* (3rd edn). Hampshire: Palgrave Macmillan

Campbell, H., Hothkiss, R., Bradshaw, N. and Poteous, M. (1998) 'Integrated Care Pathways'. *British Medical Journal*, 316 (10 January): 133–137

Clarke, J. and Copcutt, L. (1997) *Management for Nurses and Health Professionals*. Edinburgh: Churchill Livingstone

Department of Health (1989) *Working for Patients*. London: HMSO

Department of Health (1991) *The Patients' Charter*. London: HMSO

Department of Health (1998) *A First Class Service – Improving quality in the New NHS*. London: Department of Health

Department of Health (1999) *Making a Difference*. London: Department of Health

Department of Health (2000a) *An Organization With a Memory: Report of an expert group on learning from adverse events in the NHS*. London: Department of Health

Department of Health (2000b) *No Secrets: Guidance on developing and implementing multi-agency policies and procedures to protect vulnerable adults from abuse*. London: Department of Health

Department of Health (2000c) *The Care Standards Act*. London: The Stationery Office

Department of Health (2000d) *The NHS Plan: A Plan for Investment: A Plan for Reform*. London: Department of Health

Department of Health (2001a) *Building a Safer NHS for Patients: Implementing an organization with a memory*. London: Department of Health

Department of Health (2001b) *Essence of Care: Patient focused benchmarking for health care practitioners*. London: Department of Health

Department of Health (2003) The Health and Social Care Act. London: Department of Health

Department of Health (2006a) *Safety First – A report for patients, clinicians and healthcare managers*. London: Department of Health

Department of Health (2006b) The Safeguarding of Vulnerable Groups Act. London: Department of Health

Department of Health (2008) Local Government and Public Health Act. London: Department of Health

Dowding, L. and Barr, J. (2002) *Managing in Healthcare*. Harlow: Pearson Education

Irwin, P. and Fordham, J. (1995) *Evaluating the Quality of Care*. Edinburgh: Churchill Livingstone

Marr, H. and Giebing, H. (1994) *Quality Assurance in Nursing: Concepts, methods and case studies*. Oxford: Campion Press

Middleton, S., Barnett, J. and Reeves, D. (2003) *What is an Integrated Care Pathway?* Hayward Medical Communications. Available at **www.evidence-based-medicine.co.uk** (accessed 12/4/09)

Milligan, F. (2003) 'Adverse health-care events: Part 1. The nature of the problem'. *Professional Nurse*, 18 (9): 502–505

NHS Executive (1994) *The Evolution of Clinical Audit*. London: HMSO

Nursing and Midwifery Council (2009) *Registrant/client relationships and the prevention of abuse*. Available at **www.nmc-org.uk** (accessed 16/5/09)

O'Rourke, A. (2005) 'Minimising clinical risk'. *Current Paediatrics*, 15 (6): 466–472

Royal College of Nursing (2003) *Clinical Governance: A RCN resource guide.* London: RCN

Sale, D. (2005) *Understanding Clinical Governance and Quality Assurance.* Hampshire: Palgrave Macmillan

Som, C.W. (2004) 'Clinical governance: A fresh look at its definition'. *Clinical Governance: An International Journal*, 9 (2): 87–89

Useful websites

www.cppih.org/about_what.html (accessed 23/2/2009)

www.cqc.org.uk (accessed 23/02/09)

www.nice.org.uk/pdf/BestPracticeClinicalAudit.pdf (accessed 27/2/09)

www.pals.nhs.uk (accessed 27/2/09)

www.csp.org.uk (accessed 28/2/09)

www.healthcarecommission.org.uk/aboutus/whatwedo (accessed 23/2/09)

www.dh.gov.uk/en/managingyourorganisation/legalandcontractual/complaintspolicy/NHScomplaintsprocedureDH_4080897 (accessed 25/2/09)

www.library.nhs.uk/healthmanagement/viewResources.aspx?resID=267743&tabID=2908summaries=trueresultsPerPage=108sort=1 (accessed 24/2/09)

www.dh.gov.uk/en/Publicationsandstatistics/PublishedSurvey/NationalsurveyofNHSpatients/index.htm (accessed 25/2/09)

www.cqc.org.uk/aboutcqc.cfm (accessed 9/04/09)

Chapter 8

Evidence-based Practice

The aim of this chapter is to remind you about the importance of respecting research and evidence-based practice within your nursing role, both as a student and when you register with the NMC. Lindsay (2007) emphasises that practice requires students not only to perform skilfully but also to support their actions by referring to evidence.

Outcomes

On completion of this chapter you should be able to:

- review your understanding of evidence-based practice and the need to consider this when carrying out nursing care.

INTRODUCTION

Historically nursing and, specifically, clinical procedures, have been based on rituals rather than research (Dougherty and Lister, 2008) but, over the last few decades, the term 'evidence-based practice' has become common parlance within the nursing profession. Many authors have proffered definitions as to what they believe evidence-based practice involves: Ingersoll (2000, p. 152) suggests 'evidence-based nursing practice is the conscientious, explicit and judicious use of theory-derived, research-based information in making decisions about care delivery to individuals or groups of patients with consideration of individual needs and preferences'. White (1997) simplifies this by describing it as a method of problem-solving that involves identifying a clinical problem, searching the literature, evaluating the research evidence and deciding on the intervention. Dawes *et al.* (2005) believe evidence-based practice ensures that decisions on patient management are made using evidence that has been critically appraised and presented in understandable terms rather than research jargon. Finally, Hamer and Collinson (2005, p. 6) add that the 'ultimate goal of evidence-based practice is to support the practitioner in their decision making in order to eliminate the use of ineffective, inappropriate, too expensive and potentially dangerous practices'.

Notwithstanding the above definitions the central tenet of evidence-based practice is that practitioners combine their clinical or practice expertise and their knowledge of the client or patient with high-quality evidence from research (Sackett *et al.*, 1996). It is therefore an opportunity to bridge the gap between research on the one hand and practice on the other.

Figure 1 gives an example of the relationship between the three components of evidence-based practice (from Rycroft-Malone *et al.*, 2004).

EVIDENCE-BASED PRACTICE IN NURSING

In undertaking professional roles today nurses need to understand how information derived from research is turned into 'evidence' and thus informs practice. The NMC (NMC, 2008, p. 7) clearly identifies that nurses have a responsibility to 'deliver care based on the best available evidence or best practice'. The Department of Health points out that the expectations of patients can be considered as a driver for nursing practice these days – 'patients are more knowledgeable and expect to be treated as partners and equals, and have to have choices and opinions available to them' (Department of Health, 2006, p. 6).

Evidence-based practice in nursing has its roots in the evidence-based medicine movement but, in nursing, definitions based on the patient's views of effectiveness are given prominence. The RCN (1996a) emphasises this by saying:

> Evidence-based health care is rooted in the best scientific evidence and takes into account patients' views of effectiveness and clinical expertise in order to promote clinically effective services. This is essential in ensuring that health care practitioners do the things that work and are acceptable to patients, and do not do the things which don't work.
>
> (RCN, 1996a, cited in McClary and Duff, 1997, p. 31)

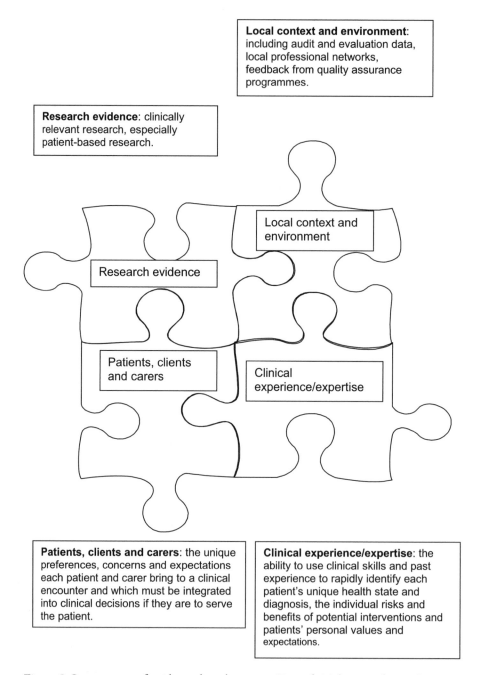

Local context and environment: including audit and evaluation data, local professional networks, feedback from quality assurance programmes.

Research evidence: clinically relevant research, especially patient-based research.

Local context and environment

Research evidence

Patients, clients and carers

Clinical experience/expertise

Patients, clients and carers: the unique preferences, concerns and expectations each patient and carer bring to a clinical encounter and which must be integrated into clinical decisions if they are to serve the patient.

Clinical experience/expertise: the ability to use clinical skills and past experience to rapidly identify each patient's unique health state and diagnosis, the individual risks and benefits of potential interventions and patients' personal values and expectations.

Figure 1 Components of evidence-based practice (Rycroft-Malone *et al.*, 2004)

The Royal College of Nursing (1996b) further states that nurses must show they are doing the right thing, in the right way, and at the right time, for the right patient. This is expanded upon by Bury and Mead (1998) and illustrated in Figure 2 from Williamson *et al.* (2008):

The right person	Was the person delivering the care competent, with the right skills and knowledge?
The right thing	Was there evidence to support the intervention, and was the patient agreeable?
The right way	Was an intervention used correctly, with correct skills and competence, or did it meet national guidelines and priorities?
The right place	Could the patient have been treated at home, or was there a more appropriate place based on specialist equipment or staff?
The right time	Was the intervention timely – would it have been more effective without a six-month wait?
The right result	Did it do what was intended?

Figure 2 'Six Rs' of clinical effectiveness (Williamson *et al.*, 2008, adapted from Bury and Mead, 1998)

Such statements by the RCN clearly highlight the importance of evidence-based practice in nursing. Parahoo (2006) points out that nurses represent the largest group of health care professionals throughout the world and spend considerably more time with patients than any other health professional group. Therefore, as a profession, nursing must build its body of knowledge on solid grounds. However, Craig and Smyth (2003) issue a note of caution to this – the huge range of settings and people that nurses work with can be detrimental to implementing evidence-based practice; the settings in which nurses work are so varied that research cannot possibly be relevant to all. So, what is the right thing and what are the choices available? Craig and Smyth (2003) believe that because of the range of settings and people with which nurses work, the concept of evidence-based practice is particularly challenging for them.

Lindsay (2007, p. 4) outlines what he considers the most important reasons for practice to be based on evidence as:

- the public no longer trusts health and social care professionals to do what is best;
- professionals are conscious of the risk of being sued and want clear evidence for their practices;
- emerging health and social care professions want to create their own evidence for their roles;
- governments demand clear evidence before funding expensive new treatments or care strategies.

There are many reasons why using evidence-based practice in nursing is important and the list below does not begin to cover them all, but is a starting point. It:

- establishes justifiable, defensible reasons for nursing actions;
- increases cost-effective practice;
- enhances clinical effectiveness;
- is a basis for assuring quality care delivery (clinical governance);
- improves the patient's experience;
- provides evidence of what does not work;
- provides evidence to support resource allocation;
- supports managing risk;
- encourages academic and professional development.

Carrying out evidence-based practice

Several authors (Williamson *et al.*, 2008; Offredy, 2006; Sackett *et al.*, 2000) suggest a sequence of events that has to take place before information can be considered 'evidence-based'. This is summarised in Figure 3.

What is evidence?

In the past, proponents of evidence-based practice have focused on research derived from quantitative methods (data collected in the form of numbers), as they were deemed the only studies worth considering; and there was little or no recognition of research gathered by qualitative means (data collected in the form of words) (Ingersoll, 2000). Dougherty and Lister (2008) believe this was worrying when, within nursing, qualitative

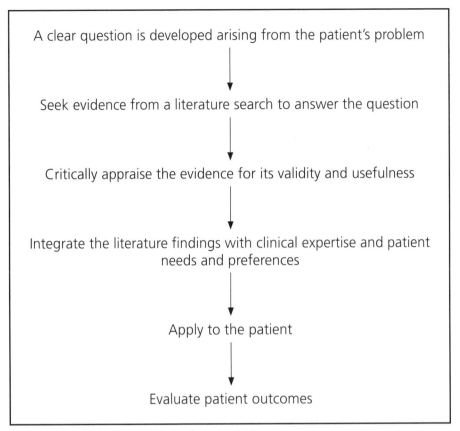

A clear question is developed arising from the patient's problem

Seek evidence from a literature search to answer the question

Critically appraise the evidence for its validity and usefulness

Integrate the literature findings with clinical expertise and patient needs and preferences

Apply to the patient

Evaluate patient outcomes

Figure 3 The sequence of evidence-based practice

research is the prevalent design used. However, this is beginning to change as, increasingly, evidence is recognised as coming from many different areas (as shown in Figure 1), with the acknowledgement that it has been subjected to testing and been found credible (Higgs *et al.*, 2008)

Credibility is key in evidence-based practice but there is little consensus about how evidence is assessed before it is used to inform practice, mainly because making such judgements about evidence is complex and difficult to achieve (Dougherty and Lister, 2008). In some instances government bodies have developed nationally accepted guidelines as a result of expert researchers undertaking research trials – examples of these are the NICE guidelines and National Service Frameworks (NSFs), which were developed to achieve consistent clinical standards across the NHS (Department of Health, 1998). In other instances some hospitals have created their own nursing guidelines where procedures are regularly reviewed and updated for example, the Royal Marsden Hospital's *Clinical Nursing Procedures* (Dougherty and Lister, 2008) and the Liverpool care pathway for the dying patient (**www.mcpil.org.uk/liverpool-care-pathway/index.htm**), and published them, thereby enabling other health care professionals and patients to benefit from their work.

Activity

Where might you obtain information about specific evidence-based practice required to deliver high-quality nursing care? Make a list of the resources available to nurses.

Critical awareness

Society's health care needs are constantly changing, which requires nurses to keep their knowledge up to date if they are to provide the best possible care to patients. It is equally the case that nurses need to challenge everyday practices to ensure they are safe for use with patients. A major part of keeping care up to date is reviewing or evaluating literature on the subject. Evaluating research always sounds rather daunting for the inexperienced but it can be broken down into a number of simple steps.

Firstly, all research needs to be reliable (truthful) and valid (transferable), but not all research is necessarily relevant or applicable (Lindsay, 2007). Evidence sought needs to be linked directly to nurses' practice, and inform that practice, thereby making it relevant and applicable. Pearson (2000) is concerned that research results do not always relate to the reality of everyday practice, an example of which is a project where the use of ordinary tap water for wound cleansing was advocated, but the study was carried out in a 'Western country' where water is 'purified', so the use of water in some countries would not be appropriate.

Secondly, nurses need to be critical of the evidence they use to inform their practice in order to enable them to decide the value or worth of a piece of research, given the purposes for which it is to be used. Hamer and Collinson (2005, p. 11) list qualities they believe are required for nurses to be 'critical', which are:

- to be questioning;
- to see more than one side of an argument;
- to be objective rather than subjective;
- to weigh evidence;
- to judge others' statements as being based on reason, evidence or

logic on the one hand or based on partial evidence, special pleading, emotion or self-interest on the other;

- to look at the meaning behind the facts;
- to identify issues arising from the facts;
- to recognise when further evidence is needed.

Thirdly, nurses need to know how to evaluate a research article. Walsh (1997) states that the decision (and ultimate accountability) lies with individual nurses to assess if the evidence they use is relevant, so therefore they need the skills to evaluate the evidence critically. Below are some hints for evaluating research articles which are taken from **www.rip.org. uk/research_resources/evaluating.asp.** Although a comprehensive guide to this process, not all pointers may be able to be addressed – it depends on the focus of the research article.

The article

The title – is it informative, interesting and to the point? i.e., does it address the question that you want answered?

The authors – what do you know about the authors? Do they have a vested interest in the conclusions of the study?

The abstract – does it summarise the main points of the study adequately and accurately? Be careful, as sometimes abstracts promise more than what is written in the rest of the paper.

Introduction – is the problem or purpose of the study clearly stated?

The questions – are they stated clearly and concisely? Do they follow logically from the problems? Are they worth answering? Are they answerable?

The literature – is the background information adequate? Does the author appear to know her/his subject? Does he/she appraise related research and authoritative statements? Or has he/she strung together citations and quotes that support her/his proposal without consideration of antagonistic arguments? Are specific theories used in order to put the study and potentially the findings into context? Does this theory seem relevant?

Relevance – is the study placed in the context of current professional knowledge? What is the potential contribution of the study to practice?

Aims – are the aims stated clearly, concisely and precisely? Are they logically related to the original questions? How were they formulated; for example, does evidence from the literature support intuition, instinct and experience? If treatment is being investigated, are the aims related to efficacy and safety?

The method

Design – is the study descriptive or experimental? Is it described adequately? Does the chosen design seem appropriate to you? A hypothesis or hypotheses is/are necessary for an experimental design. Does it/do they follow logically from the original problem and theories?

Assumptions – are any assumptions being made? Is their use explained? Are they justifiable and appropriate? Was a pilot study completed, i.e. was a questionnaire or special report pre-tested for validity and/or reliability? Were modifications made? What were they and why?

Ethical considerations – has the author considered the ethics of the proposal? Is the proposed method ethically acceptable? For example, will all service users receive the treatment/intervention they need rather than the treatment needed for the study? Will a control group be required to receive a bogus or dummy treatment of dubious efficacy?

Participants – how were people selected? Are individuals allocated to alternative treatment/intervention groups? Is this ethical? Is there an account of how each person was chosen? Were specific criteria used to include and/or exclude people in/from the study? Are they clearly stated? Is the reasoning behind them apparent and sensible?

Samples – was a specific size of sample chosen (for example, for statistical purposes)? Does it seem adequate to provide sustainable results? If the author aims to make general comments about a population on the basis of the findings, who forms this population? Is the sample representative of this population?

Data collection – is the method described adequately? Could you replicate it from the description? Are the reasons for the choice of method stated? If special report forms, assessment forms, questionnaires, or interview schedules have been used, are copies provided with the paper or is an address given for copies?

Analysis – is the method of analysis understandable? Have statistical tests been used? Are reasons for choice given that explain their appropriateness? Do you understand and accept the explanation?

Results – are results intelligible enough for you to interpret them and draw your own conclusions? Are they relevant to the stated problem? Does your background knowledge and common sense indicate that they are realistic and feasible? Are 'raw' data given, or only proportions, percentages, etc., after manipulation? Are histograms, pie charts and other graphic representations explained? Are the tables helpful? If results are based on responses to a questionnaire or interview schedule, what is the response rate? Are statistical results included? Are they meaningful? Is the statistical probability of results by chance included? Is it appropriate?

Discussion – are the results interpreted in relation to the original question(s)? Are the original questions answered? Have the aims been fulfilled? Does the author discuss any weaknesses in the methodology and factors that may have affected validity or reliability? For example: should selection of sample be discussed? If criteria of inclusion and exclusion need clarification, is the explanation acceptable? Should the advantages and disadvantages of the method of data collection be discussed? Are they? Have you noticed anything that was omitted? Has the author referred to it or ignored it? Have the findings been related to the existing body of knowledge and relevant theory? Are the clinical implications discussed? Was the project funded? By whom? Might the results be biased because of the interests of the financing body?

Conclusions – how do they compare (or contrast) with the conclusions you drew from your interpretation of the results? Do they relate logically to the results?

Recommendations – are the recommended changes self-evident from the reported results? Could you attempt to implement them, and should you? Is this study an end in itself, or does it suggest further research?

References – is the length of the list more impressive than its quality? Are any references conspicuous by their absence?

Activity

- Go to the Research Mindedness website **www.resmind.swap. ac.uk** and click on the section 'are you research minded?', and undertake the self-evaluation questionnaire.
- Now find a research article in any nursing journal and review it taking into account the above hints.

Clinical effectiveness (does it work?)

The term 'evidence-based practice' is often linked with clinical effectiveness. Williamson *et al.* (2008) believe clinical effectiveness is concerned with using treatments or care that have been shown to work, and it is important that what nurses do is effective because 'the NHS is a publicly funded service and it would be financially wasteful, pointless and immoral . . . to be using particular clinical interventions if they were not known to be effective' (Williamson *et al.*, 2008, p. 82).

The link between evidence-based practice and clinical effectiveness can be seen in the RCN's (1996b, p.1) definition of clinical effectiveness: 'applying the best available knowledge, derived from research, clinical expertise and patient preferences, to achieve optimum processes and outcomes of care for patients' – a definition not dissimilar to that of evidence-based practice.

McClarey and Duff (1997) believe clinical effectiveness has three distinct parts – again not very different from evidence-based practice.

- **Obtaining evidence** – from research, either published in journals or available on databases; from national level studies based on research, for example, clinical guidelines, systematic reviews or national standards.
- **Implementing the evidence** – by changing practice to include the research evidence and where possible locally adapting national standards or guidelines.
- **Evaluating the impact of the changed practice** – and readjusting practice as necessary, usually through clinical audit and patient feedback.

Clinical effectiveness is also linked to clinical governance (see Chapter 7 on 'Quality assurance'). Solomon (2003) states that clinical-governance initiatives introduced by the government (Department of Health, 1998) aim to ensure that care provided is of high quality and has effective outcomes. These outcomes are achieved by employing the principles of evidence-based practice. Colyer and Kamath (1999, cited in Palfreyman *et al.*, 2003) add the economic benefits of evidence-based practice to their definition as they believe the overall purpose of evidence-based practice is to provide effective health care within the limited resources available. The Department of Health endorses this by saying demonstrating clinical and cost effectiveness is a key goal for the NHS (Department of Health, 1995, 1997) and one means of achieving this is evidence-based practice.

Factors affecting the implementation of evidence-based practice

As indicated throughout this chapter the use of evidence-based practice is critical to nurses, whether they be students or registered professionals. However, Dougherty and Lister (2008) point out that, on the whole, delivering evidence-based care can be demanding and needs determination and time. Reasons for nurses not engaging in this practice have been cited by many authors, perhaps best summarised by Ciliska *et al.* (2001, p. 520) who say: 'barriers [to evidence-based practice] occur when time, access to journal articles, search skills, critical appraisal skills, and understanding of the language used in research are lacking'.

Other authors have also highlighted difficulties in engaging nurses in research and evidence-based practice (Gerrish and Lacey, 2006; Palfreyman *et al.*, 2003; Craig and Smyth, 2003) – some explanations for this are listed below.

- The nature of evidence:
  - lack of clinically relevant research in nursing;
  - what do you do if there is no evidence?;
  - tension between evidence and practice – where research unequivocally says 'X' works, and it doesn't;
  - research is applied in a set of experimental conditions and cannot be reproduced in real-life settings.

- How evidence is communicated:
  - often published in academic journals, rather than professional journals which clinical nurses are more likely to read;
  - limited places at conferences where up-to-date information is presented;
  - the language of research is sometimes a barrier;
  - researchers fail to draw out the implications of their research for practice.

- Knowledge and skills of individual nurses:
  - nurses do not have the knowledge and skills to access and appraise research information;
  - changing practice is exhausting – how often are nurses asked to do this?;
  - changing practice involves accepting that you may have ceased to be right, and maybe for some time.

- Organisational barriers:
  - time, heavy clinical workloads;
  - lack of authority and support to implement findings;
  - implementing research in one area of practice may disrupt other areas.

Finally, Lindsay (2007) reminds nurses that evidence is not only used to 'change' practice, it can also be used to support existing practice, while

Walsh (1997) believes research needs to be done by some, facilitated by others, and 'implemented' by all.

Activity

Choose a nursing duty and explore the literature about it. Then compare your findings with the practice you observe in your clinical area. Do they differ and, if so, what would you do about it?

Further reading

This chapter does not seek to discuss research methodologies, nor how to seek out literature – there are many academic textbooks that can help you with that. One such is Lindsay, B. (2007) *Understanding Research and Evidence-Based Practice*. Exeter: Reflect Press.

REFERENCES

Bury, T. and Mead, J. (1998) *Evidence-based Health Care: A practical guide for therapists.* Oxford: Butterworth-Heinemann

Ciliska, D., Pinelli, J., DiCenso, A. and Cullum, N. (2001) 'AACN clinical issues'. *Advanced Practice in Acute and Critical Care*, 12 (4): 520–528

Colyer, H. and Kamath, P. (1999) 'Evidence-based practice. A philosophical and political analysis: Some matters for consideration by professional practitioners'. *Journal of Advanced Nursing*, 29 (1): 188–193, cited in Palfreyman, S., Tod, S. and Doyle, J. (2003) 'An integrated approach to evidence-based practice'. *The Foundation of Nursing Studies Dissemination Series*, 1 (9): 1–4

Craig, J. and Smyth, R. (2003) *The Evidence-Based Practice Manual.* Edinburgh: Churchill Livingstone

Dawes, M., Davies, P., Gray, A., Mant, J., Seers, K. and Snowball, R. (2005) *Evidence-based Practice: A primer for healthcare professionals* (2nd edn). Edinburgh: Elsevier Churchill Livingstone

Department of Health (1995) *Research and Development: Towards an evidence-based health service.* London: HMSO

Department of Health (1997) *The New NHS: Modern and dependable.* London: HMSO

Department of Health (1998) *A First Class Service: Quality in the new NHS*. London: HMSO

Department of Health (2006) *Modernising Nursing Careers*. London: Department of Health

Dougherty, L. and Lister, S. (2008) *The Royal Marsden Hospital Manual of Clinical Nursing Procedures: Student Edition*. Chichester: Wiley-Blackwell

Gerrish, K. and Lacey, A. (2006) *The Research Process in Nursing*. Oxford: Blackwell

Hamer, S. and Collinson, G. (2005) *Achieving Evidence-Based Practice* (2nd edn). Edinburgh: Baillière Tindall

Higgs, J., Jones, M., Loftus, S. and Christensen, N. (2008) *Clinical Reasoning in the Health Professions* (3rd edn). Oxford: Butterworth Heinemann

Ingersoll, G. (2000) 'Evidence-based nursing: What it is and what it isn't'. *Nursing Outlook*, 48 (4): 151–152

Lindsay, B. (2007) *Understanding Research and Evidence-based Practice*. Exeter: Reflect Press

McClarey, M. and Duff, L. (1997) 'Clinical effectiveness and evidence-based practice'. *Nursing Standard*, 11 (51): 31–35

Nursing and Midwifery Council (2008) *The Code: Standards of conduct, performance and ethics for nurses and midwives*. London: NMC

Offredy, M. (2006) 'Evidence-based practice', cited in Peate, I. (2006) *Becoming a Nurse In The 21st Century*. Chichester: John Wiley and Sons

Palfreyman, S., Tod, S. and Doyle, J. (2003) 'An integrated approach to evidence-based practice'. *The Foundation of Nursing Studies Dissemination Series*, 1 (9): 1–4

Parahoo, K. (2006) *Nursing Research Principles, Process and Issues*. Basingstoke: Palgrave Macmillan

Pearson, M. (2000) 'Making a difference through research: How nurses can turn the vision into reality (editorial)'. *Nursing Times Research*, 5 (2): 85–86

Royal College of Nursing (1996a) *The Royal College of Nursing Clinical Effectiveness Initiative – A Strategic Framework*. London: RCN, cited in McClarey, M. and Duff, L. (1997) 'Clinical effectiveness and evidence-based practice'. *Nursing Standard*, 11 (51): 31–35

Royal College of Nursing (1996b) *Clinical Effectiveness*. London: RCN

Rycroft-Malone, J., Seers, K., Titchen, A., Harvey, G., Kitson, A. and McCormack, B. (2004) 'What counts as evidence in evidence-based practice'. *Journal of Advanced Nursing*, 47: 81–90

Sackett, D., Rosenberg, W. and Gray, J., Haynes, R. and Richardson, W. (1996) 'Evidence-based medicine: What it is and what it isn't'. *British Medical Journal*, 312: 71–72

Sackett, D., Richardson, S., Rosenberg, W. and Haynes. R. (2000) *Evidence-Based Medicine: How to teach and practice* (2nd edn). London: Churchill Livingstone

Solomon, J. (2003) 'Eating and drinking', cited in Holland, K., Jenkins, J., Solomon, J. and Whittam, S. (eds) *Roper, Logan and Tierney Model in Practice*. Edinburgh: Churchill Livingstone

Walsh, M. (1997) 'How nurses perceive barriers to research implementation'. *Nursing Standard*, 8 (11): 25-29

White, S. (1997) 'Evidence-based practice and nursing: The new panacea?' *British Journal of Nursing*, Feb 13-26; 6 (3): 175–178

Williamson, G., Jenkinson, T. and Proctor-Childs, T. (2008) *Nursing in Contemporary Healthcare Practice*. Exeter: Learning Matters

Useful websites

www.resmind.swap.ac.uk
www.library.nhs.uk/Default.aspx
http://ebn.bmj.com
http://clinicalevidence.bmj.com/ceweb/index.jsp
www.cochranelibrary.com
www.mcpcil.org.uk/liverpool_care_pathway
www.nice.org.uk

Chapter 9

Health Promotion

Nurses have a key role in promoting health to the people they care for and the wider community. Therefore, the aim of this chapter is to briefly explore the concept of health promotion and public health in the context of health care in the United Kingdom.

Outcomes

On completion of this chapter you should be able to:

- briefly explain the concept of health;

- identify the various approaches to health promotion;

- appraise the influence of different factors on an individual's health related behaviour;

- recognise current government strategies with regard to health promotion and public health.

INTRODUCTION

Before considering specific aspects of health promotion it is important to have some understanding of how an individual within your care might define and prioritise health. Such knowledge can help you as a nurse to tailor interventions to the needs of the person, and to enhance the relevance and success of those interventions. The following are some definitions of health offered in the literature.

> A state of complete physical, mental and social well being and not merely the absence of disease and infirmity.
>
> (WHO, 1946/84, cited in Naidoo and Wills, 2000, p.6)

. . . freedom from medically defined disease and disability.
(Ewles and Simnett, 1992, p. 6)

Health and disease cannot be defined merely in terms of anatomical, physiological or mental attributes. The real measure is the ability of the individual to function in a manner acceptable to himself and to the group of which he/she is part.
(Dubos, 1959, cited in Seedhouse, 1986, p. 41)

Health designates the ability to adapt to changing environments, to growing up and to ageing, to healing when damaged, to suffering and to the peaceful expectation of death.
(Illich, 1977, p. 273)

By health I mean the power to live a full, adult, living, breathing life, in close contact with what I love . . . I want to be all that I am capable of becoming.
(Mansfield, 1927, cited in Stead, 1977, p. 278)

Activity

Take a few minutes to consider how close or otherwise the quotations above may be to your own definition of health.

You should not be concerned if your definition of health differs from those above as it is important to remember that there are no right or wrong definitions. The following factors should also be taken into account.

- **Health means different things to different people** – that is, it is individually defined and we all have our own personal list of priorities. This has implications for health promotion in as much as health care professionals should work with the patient/client's priorities and perceptions of health, rather than their own, if they are to maximise effective/positive outcomes.
- **Perceptions of health may be relative** – to age, life situation, life experiences, cultural influences, etc. Our health priorities will be influenced by these factors and will inevitably change through life, thereby re-emphasising the 'individuality' of health perceptions.

- **Health and illness may coexist** – for some, health is an ideal state to aim at, whereas others emphasise the need for realism/pragmatism.
- **Health can also be linked to a sense of well-being** – that is, 'the feel-good factor'.
- **Health care can be viewed holistically** – Aggleton (1990) stresses that health does not exist purely within the individual: there are elements outside the individual that also constitute health. They don't just influence health, they are 'dimensions' of health itself and therefore they include not only emotional, psychological, physical and sexual dimensions but also, in a wider context, social, environmental and spiritual dimensions. Individuals put emphasis on different aspects according to personal priorities.

Activity

Becoming a student of nursing may initially involve significant changes to your life. Within the dimensions of health identified above, what do you perceive as the priorities for your own health during this time?

Understanding the factors that may affect your health or sense of well-being may assist in your maintaining a positive health status while working in a health care environment.

Further reading

Further reading around lay concepts of health can be accessed at **www.answers.com/topic/lay-concepts-of-health-and-illness** or **www.uta.fi/laitokset/tsph/health/citizens/lay1.html** Both briefly explore some of the theoretical underpinnings of lay concepts of health.

HEALTH PROMOTION

In 1989 the Department of Health recommended that health promotion should be a recognised part of health care and that all practitioners (including nurses) should develop skills in, and utilise every opportunity for, health promotion. Subsequent legislation and policy, for example, *Saving Lives: Our Healthier Nation* (Department of Health, 1999) and *Choosing Health: Making healthy choices easier* (Department of Health 2004), has reinforced this recommendation.

Although Seedhouse (1997) suggests that the area of health promotion is confused, poorly articulated and devoid of a clear philosophy, there are a considerable number of definitions of health promotion to be found in the literature. They include the following.

> Process of enabling people to increase control over and to improve their health.
>
> (WHO, 1986, p. 1)

> Attempts to persuade, cajole or otherwise influence individuals to alter their lifestyle.
>
> (Gott and O'Brien, 1990, p.30)

> The balanced enhancement of physical, mental, and social facets of positive health, coupled with the prevention of physical, mental and social ill health.
>
> (Downie *et al.*, 1998, p. 26)

> Health promotion is about raising the health status of individuals and communities . . . by promotion in the health context we mean improving health; advancing, supporting, encouraging and placing it higher on personal and public agendas.
>
> (Ewles and Simnett, 1992, p. 19)

> An approach and philosophy of care which reflects awareness of the multiplicity of factors which affect health and which encourages everyone to value independence and individual choice.
>
> (Wilson-Barnett and Macleod, 1993,
> cited in Naidoo and Wills, 2000, p. 72)

These definitions overall reflect the current emphasis of health promotion. That is, it is about a range of activities involving individuals, communities, professionals, government, statutory and voluntary organisations.

Approaches to health promotion

Naidoo and Wills (2000) identify five different approaches to health promotion within the UK. They are:

- medical or preventive;
- behaviour change;
- educational;
- empowerment/client-centred;
- social change.

Medical approach

This approach focuses on freedom from medically defined disease and disability with the use of medical procedures to prevent or improve ill health (prevention, compliance-detection and treatment). It is often identified as having the three levels of intervention:

- **primary prevention** – (preventing the onset of disease);
- **secondary prevention** – (preventing progression of disease);
- **tertiary prevention** – (preventing recurrence of illness and reducing effects of illness).

Naidoo and Wills (2000) suggest this approach is popular because:

- it uses scientific methods such as epidemiology;
- in the short term, prevention and early detection of disease are cheaper than treatment (but not always in the long term);
- it is an expert-led, top-down intervention;
- there have been many successes, for example the worldwide eradication of smallpox.

Examples of intervention include: risk education (for example, stop smoking) immunisation programmes, screening programmes, rehabilitation, and palliative care.

Behaviour change approach

This persuasive approach aims to encourage change in attitudes and behaviour so that people adopt a 'healthier lifestyle' (often as defined by the health promoter) which, in turn, should improve health. This approach puts the responsibility for good health back on the individual, thereby suggesting that if people do not take responsible action to look after themselves then they are to blame for the consequences. It is similar to the medical approach in that it is an expert-led, top-down approach that, according to Naidoo and Wills (2000, p. 96) 'reinforces the divide between the expert who knows how to improve health and the general public who need education and advice'.

Examples of intervention include: campaigns to encourage people to stop smoking, eat a healthier diet, improve exercise levels and not to drink and drive.

Educational approach

This involves the provision of information and education to enable an individual to make informed decisions. Unlike the behaviour approach, its intention is not to persuade or motivate change in a particular direction but, by increasing knowledge, to facilitate voluntary choice.

Examples of intervention include: provision of leaflets, booklets, etc., group discussions or one-to-one counselling.

Empowerment/client-centred approach

This approach involves addressing only those issues and concerns that are identified by the client themselves and then enabling them to gain the skills and confidence to resolve or act upon those concerns. This can involve both self-empowerment and, in a wider context, community empowerment. Unlike the other approaches, this is a client-centred approach that is aimed at increasing people's control over their own lives. According to Ewles and Simnett (1999), the process of empowering involves altering how people feel about themselves by improving both their self-awareness and self-esteem. It includes helping them to think critically about their values and belief system and it is about having the resources available that enable an individual to make real and free choices.

Scriven and Orme (2001) also note that, in addition to gathering appropriate knowledge and understanding regarding the implications of health actions and having a positive attitude to relevant health-related behaviours, individuals must also believe that they have the ability to carry out these actions. The nurse's role in the process of empowering the individual includes:

- utilising good communication skills (including counselling skills);
- facilitation of decision-making through exploring the client/patient's existing beliefs, attitudes, values and skills;
- providing information;

- negotiating action plan/s;
- providing ongoing support.

(Scriven and Orme, 2001)

Examples of interventions will depend on the individual's/community's needs relevant to their concerns, but they could be as diverse as developing a care plan with a patient to supporting the development of an action group in the community.

Societal change approach

This approach involves political and societal action to change the physical, social and economic environment to enable the individual to choose a healthier lifestyle.

Examples of intervention include: policy, campaigns and legislation, for example, banning smoking in public places.

Further reading

Further information on these approaches can be accessed at: **www.patient.co.uk/showdoc/16** offers a range of information on health promotion issues and links to other relevant websites. **www.healthscotland.com**, **www.pubmedcentral.nih.gov/ articlerender.fcgi?artid=1117900** and **www.healthpromotion.ie** provide information relevant to their specific areas.

THEORIES/MODELS USED IN HEALTH PROMOTION

The main focus of health promotion over the past 20 years has been on modifying those aspects of an individual's behaviour that are known to impact on health. Understanding why people behave in a certain way and how they can be supported to continue chosen positive health behaviours is central to self-empowerment.

There are a number of theories and models that can be linked to the practice of health promotion, which attempt to explain the influence of different factors on an individual's health behaviour. These include: the Stages of Change Model (Prochaska and DiClemente, 1984) and the Health Belief Model (Rosenstock, 1966; Becker, 1974).

Stages of Change Model (Transtheoretical Model)

Originally developed in the late 1970s and early 1980s by Prochaska and DiClemente, this model seeks to identify a cycle or stages of change that an individual may pass through when changing health behaviour. The theory behind this model is that behaviour change does not all happen at one time. Rather, individuals tend to move forward, at their own rate, through a number of stages on their way to successful behaviour change. Each individual needs to decide internally, for themselves, when a stage is completed and when it is time to move onto the next stage. These stages do not necessarily just follow each other; individuals tend to move back and forth between stages, and relapse to a prior stage is always possible.

The stages of change

- **Pre-contemplation** – in this stage, the person may be unaware or barely aware that there is a problem, the cons outweigh the pros and they may be defensive towards other people's efforts to effect change in their behaviour.
- **Contemplation** – the person begins to acknowledge that there may be a problem. They are becoming more aware of the personal consequences of their behaviour, are considering change, though not quite ready or ambivalent about it, but are more open to receiving information and education.
- **Preparation** – the person has made a commitment to make change, they are beginning to gather information, set goals and may be developing plans and strategies (for example by buying a book on weight loss or enquiring about stop smoking support groups).
- **Action** – this is the stage where the person has resolved to change and has committed themselves to that process by actively taking the steps deemed necessary to effect that change. The amount of time spent in this stage varies (for example, as little as a few hours in the case of giving up smoking or losing weight). The person tends to be more receptive to receiving help and is more likely to seek support from others (a very important element for practice).
- **Maintenance** – the person continues to maintain the change in behaviour and prevent relapse. They remain aware that what they are striving for is personally worthwhile and meaningful, and they constantly reformulate the rules of their lives while acquiring new skills to deal with and prevent a return to their previous behaviour.
- **Relapse** – on the way to permanent change of behaviour many people experience relapse. The person may have consciously changed their minds or merely slipped back into old behaviour patterns. Personal feelings of discouragement and failure are often associated with this stage and these feelings can impact significantly upon the person's

self-esteem and self-confidence. This needs to be taken into account when encouraging restart of the process at the preparation or action stage.

(Prochaska and DiClemente, 1984; MacQueen *et al.*, 1999)

An example of this model could be as follows:

Pre-contemplation – the individual has not considered that they are at risk and need to use condoms.

Contemplation – the individual becomes aware of the risk and subsequent need to use condoms.

Preparation – the individual begins to think about using condoms in the coming months.

Action – the individual uses condoms consistently (for less than six months).

Maintenance – the individual continues to use condoms consistently.

Relapse – the individual may begin to use condoms less consistently or discontinue use.

The Health Belief Model

According to Roden (2004), the Health Belief Model (HBM) has been thoroughly evaluated, received empirical support and is considered to be one of the most influential models in health promotion. Initially developed in the 1950s by social psychologists Hochbaum, Rosenstock and Kegals to explain the lack of public participation in health screening and preventive programmes, it was later extended by Becker (1974) and Becker and Maiman (1975) to include all preventive health actions and illness behaviours plus screening behaviours.

The model attempts to explore what makes people take preventive action. It suggests that behaviour, motivation and goal-setting are governed by the key factors:

- the individual's perception of the value of the health goal;
- belief that a specific health action will result in prevention or relief from illness.

Within these there are four specific dimensions.

1 **Perceived susceptibility** – the feeling of vulnerability to a given condition (must have an incentive to change).

2 **Perceived severity** – feelings about the seriousness of the threat of illness (feeling threatened by current behaviour).
3 **Perceived benefits** – belief in the benefits of the action (feel the change would be beneficial and have few adverse effects).
4 **Perceived barriers** – balancing the perceived advantages against the disadvantages/obstacles to the proposed action (feel competent to carry out the change).

With this model certain triggers prompt an individual to make a decision to do something positive about their health. The triggers to action can be internal, for example concerns about their own health or a relative's or friend's illness, or external, where they are responding to outside influences such as, for example, the media, family, friends or the social environment. The individual then goes through the following thought process.

* They begin by recognising a problem, consider it and relate it to their personal circumstances.
* They weigh up the cost and benefits of doing or not doing something about it.
* They decide on a course of action (making a change or continuing as before) according to their personal beliefs about health – their beliefs about health are influenced by their cultural and social environment and personal experiences, which shape their attitude.
    (Becker, 1974; Becker and Haiman, 1975; Naidoo and Wills, 2000)

An example relating to the use of this model could be:

* **perceived susceptibility** – someone close to me dies of lung cancer;
* **perceived severity** – I do get a cough quite often – particularly in the mornings;
* **perceived benefits** – it would save a lot of money if I did give up smoking, relatives and friends would be pleased and my cough should disappear;
* **perceived barriers** – I have been smoking a long time and life is quite stressful – I need a cigarette to help me cope. I know I will find it hard without support;
* **decision** – I will try to give up smoking but must join a group to help me.

Further reading

For further reading on the Health Belief Model and Stages of Change Model and on other relevant models like, for example, the Theory of Reasoned Action and social learning theory, access a general search engine such as Google and type in 'models and theories in health promotion' or the individual name of the model you wish to explore further.

HEALTH PROMOTION POLICY

According to Naidoo and Wills (2000), health promotion has enjoyed varying levels of government support throughout the twentieth century. The extent of this support and its nature has generally varied, as you would expect, according to the political ideology of the government in power.

The current initiative in England is *Saving Lives: Our Healthier Nation* (Department of Health, 1999). This White Paper, coupled with *Reducing Health Inequalities: An action report* (Department of Health, 1998) sets out a 10-year strategy for promoting good health and tackling poor health within the UK population. The two overriding aims are to:

1 Improve the health of the population as a whole by increasing the length of life and the number of years people spend free from illness.
2 Improve the health of the worst off in society and to narrow the health gap between the better and worst off.

(Department of Health, 1999)

Improving the health of the population

Here the strategy has focused on setting targets aimed at reducing death rates in four main priority areas.

1 **Cancer** – the target is to reduce the death rate from cancer in people under 75 by at least one-fifth (approx. 100,000 lives). This is to be achieved by taking action to reduce the main causes of cancer in the UK. Thus action has included promoting a reduction of tobacco smoking and encouraging an increase in the uptake of a diet rich in cereals, fruit and vegetables. Cessation-of-smoking clinics have

been established, tobacco advertising has been banned and healthy schools programmes and healthy living centres have been set up to offer support and advice on healthy diets, etc. Early recognition of cancers is promoted through screening programmes such as cervical and breast screening. When cancer has been diagnosed, efforts have been made to try to reduce fragmentation regarding the provision and quality of services across the UK. This has included the publication of the National Service Framework for Cancer.

2   **Coronary heart disease and stroke** – the target is to reduce the death rate from coronary heart disease and stroke and related diseases in people under 75 years by at least two-fifths (approx. 200,000 lives). This is to be achieved by promoting a reduction in tobacco smoking and alcohol intake, encouraging people to eat a healthier diet, take more exercise and control their body weight. In an effort to reduce variations in health care and improve service provision, the National Service Framework for Coronary Heart Disease has set national standards and defined service models for health promotion, disease prevention, diagnosis, treatment, rehabilitation and care across the UK.

3   **Accidents** – the target is to reduce death rates from accidents by at least one-fifth (approx. 12,000 lives). This is to be achieved by the introduction of initiatives aimed at making the wider environment safer using, for example, traffic calming measures, speed and traffic management policies, safer playgrounds, road safety training and compulsory child restraints in cars for children. In the home people are encouraged to adopt safer behaviour by, for example, ensuring medication is out of the reach of children and promoting the prevention of falls.

4   **Mental health** – the target is to reduce the death rate from suicide and undetermined injury by at least one-fifth (approx. 4,000 lives). This is to be achieved by promoting good mental health and reducing risk, mainly by strengthening support systems for those at risk – including the unemployed, young isolated mothers and the recently bereaved or divorced. Reduction-in-suicides initiatives include controlling the amount of some drugs that can be bought over the counter (for example, paracetamol), support for those at high risk of suicide and the setting up of specialist mental health helplines through NHS Direct. The National Service Framework for Mental Health sets out national standards and service models and an organisational framework for providing integrated services and commissioning services.

(Department of Health, 1999)

Essence of Care

In further support of the move away from treating ill health to encouraging the promotion of healthier life choices when providing patient care, the government published, in March 2006, a new set of Essence of Care Benchmarks, that is, *Benchmarks for Promoting Health*.

Benchmarks for Promoting Health

Agreed person outcome: Everyone will be supported to make healthier choices for themselves and others (see Figure 1).

Further reading

Further information about *Essence of Care* can be obtained from Chapter 7 on 'Quality assurance' (page 129) and information about these benchmarks can be found at:
www.dh.gov.uk/en/Publicationsandstatistics/Publications/
PublicationsPolicyAndGuidance/DH_4005475

Improving the health of the worst off in society

It is well documented (for example by Black *et al.*, 1980; Acheson, 1998) that health inequality in the United Kingdom is widespread, with the most disadvantaged in society suffering the most from poor health. It is now acknowledged by the government that to improve many people's health there needs to be management and resolution of the underlying causes of ill health such as social and economic deprivation and social exclusion. The government's aim here therefore relates to policies and initiatives to tackle the wider underlying causes of ill health in the UK.

The next stage

In the ethos of social justice a commission on social determinants of health was set up by the World Health Organisation (WHO) in 2005 to gather together the evidence on what can be done to promote health equity, and to foster a global movement to achieve it. Following international collaboration (including the UK) of policymakers, researchers and civil society from countries at all levels of income and development, the commission published its report *Closing the Gap in a Generation – Health equity through action on the social determinants of health* in

Factor	Benchmark of best practice
Empowerment and informed choice	Individuals, groups and communities are helped to make positive decisions on personal health and well-being
Education for practitioners	Practitioners have and use their knowledge and skills to promote health
Assessment of health promotion needs	Individuals, groups and communities are able to identify their health promotion needs
Opportunities for health promotion	Every appropriate contact is used to enable individuals, groups and communities to find ways to maintain or improve their health and well-being
Engagement	Individuals, groups and communities are actively involved in health promotion planning and actions
Partnership	Health promotion is undertaken in partnership with others using a variety of expertise and experiences
Access and accessibility	People have access to health promoting information, services and/or support that meets their individual needs and circumstances
Environment	Individuals, groups, communities and agencies influence and create environments that promote people's health and well-being
Outcomes of promoting health	Health promoting activity has a sustainable effect that improves public health

Figure 1: *Benchmarks for Promoting Health* (Department of Health, 2006, p. 2)

August 2008. The overarching recommendations and actions identified by the commission are to:

- **improve the conditions of daily life** – the circumstances in which people are born, grow, live, work and age;
- **tackle the inequitable distribution of power, money and resources** – the structural drivers of those conditions of daily life – globally, national and locally;
- **measure the problem, evaluate the action** – expand the knowledge base, develop a workforce that is trained in the social determinants of health and raise public awareness about the social determinants of health (WHO, 2008, p. 10).

Since the commission started its work, several countries and agencies have become 'partners' seeking to 'frame policies and programmes, across the whole of society, that influence the social determinants of health and improve health equity' (WHO, 2008, p. 3). As the UK is one of those partners, future policy will inevitably be linked to the principles and actions of the report.

Public health

The public health agenda makes up the final strand of the government's 10-year health strategy and is clearly linked to the four main priority areas previously outlined. Public health is concerned with improving the health of the population, rather than treating the diseases of individual patients. The official definition of public health adopted by the government is: 'the science and art of preventing disease, prolonging life, and promoting health through the organised efforts of society' (Acheson, 1988, cited Cowley, 2002, p. 197).

In 2004 the government, following extensive consultation, published its plans on how the public health agenda would progress in England. The Public Health White Paper, *Choosing Health: Making healthy choices easier* (Department of Health, 2004), outlined three key principles that were to underpin the strategy. They were:

- **informed choice** – including providing credible and trustworthy information to help people to make informed choices;
- **personalisation** – including support and services to be tailored to meet the realities of people's lives;
- **working together** – involving partnerships across the NHS, local government, the independent sector, voluntary sector, businesses, local communities, the media, religious groups, etc.

A set of priorities was established that were to be targeted through government, the media and locally based campaigns and initiatives and encouragement of individual responsibility in the identified areas. The priorities were identified as:

- reducing the numbers of people who smoke;
- reducing obesity and improving diet and nutrition;
- increasing exercise;
- encouraging and supporting sensible drinking;
- improving sexual health;
- improving mental health.

(These reflect the targets set out in the Health of the Nation document (DH 1999)).

Social marketing

Linked to the public health delivery systems is the social marketing approach. The term 'social marketing' was first used in the 1970s and refers to the 'application of marketing to the solution of social and health problems' (**www.dh.gov.uk/en/publichealth/Choosinghealth**). According to the National Social Marketing Centre, there are six features and concepts that are key to understanding social marketing.

1 **Customer or consumer orientation** – relates to understanding the knowledge base and attitudes and beliefs of the customer and the social context in which they live.
2 **Behaviour and behavioural goals** – relates to understanding existing behaviour and the key influences upon it, in conjunction with developing clear behavioural goals.
3 **'Intervention mix' and 'marketing mix'** – relates to utilising a variety of different interventions or methods to achieve a particular behavioural goal.
4 **Audience segmentation** – relates to clarity of audience focus using audience segmentation (dividing or grouping based on common characteristics related to behaviour) to target effectively.
5 **'Exchange'** – relates to understanding what is expected of people and the actual cost to them.
6 **'Competition'** – relates to understanding factors that impact on people and that compete for their time and attention.

www.nsms.org.uk

Further reading

Further information on social marketing can be obtained from **www.nsms.org.uk** and **www.dh.gov.uk/en/Publichealth/ Choosinghealth/DH_066342** and by using a general search engine such as Google.

Nurses and, in particular, specialist community public health nurses (health visitors), have an important part to play in the public health agenda. In order to achieve this, the government has sought to modernise the health visitor's role to enable them to build on their work with individuals, families and communities to further improve health and tackle health inequalities

A considerable number of the strategies and initiatives outlined in both *Saving Lives: Our Healthier Nation* (Department of Health, 1999) and *Choosing Health: Making healthy choices easier* (Department of Health, 2004) have now been introduced. How successful they have been is still the subject of ongoing research.

National Institute for Health and Clinical Excellence (NICE)

NICE provides public health guidance for staff working in the NHS, private and voluntary sectors and for local authorities. In general, nurses and other health care professionals are expected to follow this guidance, unless the recommendations are not deemed suitable for someone because of his or her medical condition, general health, wishes or a combination of these. There are two types of NICE public health guidance.

- **Public health intervention guidance** – recommendations on types of activities provided by local organisations that may help reduce people's risk of developing a disease or condition or help maintain a healthy lifestyle;
- **Public health programme guidance** – covers broader action for the promotion of good health and the prevention of ill health – the guidance may focus on a topic, for example smoking; on a particular population, for example older people; or on a particular setting, for example the workplace.

www.nice.org.uk

Further reading

If you wish to explore issues around current public health policy, a good starting point could be:
www.nice.org.uk for further details regarding public health guidance.
www.dh.gov.uk/en/Aboutus/MinistersandDepartmentLeaders/ChiefMedicalOfficer/index.htm and select from the index 'On the State of Public Health: Annual Report of the Chief Medical Officer', which highlights current health challenges that face the UK and details the progress made in key action areas.
Public Health in England (2008/9) available from www.dh.gov.uk, which provides an overview of current and regional public health, international comparisons and links to further relevant information.
Specific information on Scotland, Wales and Northern Ireland can be obtained from www.scotpho.org.uk/home/home.asp, www.wales.nhs.uk and follow links for public health, www.dhsspsni.gov.uk and again follow public health links.

REFERENCES

Acheson, D. (1998) *Report of the Independent Inquiry into Inequalities in Health*. London: HMSO

Aggleton, P. (1990) *Health*. London: Routledge

Becker, M.H. (ed.) (1974) *The Health Belief Model and Personal Health Behaviour*. New Jersey: Thorofare

Becker, M.H. and Maiman, L.A. (1975) 'Socio-behavioural determinants of compliance with medical care recommendations'. *Medical Care* (xiii): 10–24

Black, D., Morris, J., Smith, C. and Townsend, P. (1980) *Inequalities in Health: Report of a research working group*. London: Department of Health and Social Security

Cowley, S. (ed.) (2002) *Public Health in Policy and Practice: A Sourcebook for Health Visitors and Community Nurses*. London: Baillière Tindall

Department of Health (1998) *Reducing Health Inequalities: An action report*. London: The Stationery Office

Department of Health (1999) *Saving Lives: Our healthier nation*. London: The Stationery Office

Department of Health (2004) *Choosing Health: Making healthy choices easier.* London: The Stationery Office

Department of Health (2006) E*ssence of Care: Benchmarks for promoting health.* London: Department of Health

Downie, R.S., Tannahill, C. and Tannahill, A. (1998) *Health Promotion – Models and values.* Oxford: Oxford University Press

Ewles, L. and Simnett, I. (1992) *Promoting Health: A Practical Guide* (2nd edn). London: Scutari Press

Ewles, L. and Simnett, I. (1999) *Promoting Health: A Practical Guide* (4th edn). London: Ballière Tindall

Gott, M. and O'Brien, M. (1990) 'Attitudes and belief in health promotion'. *Nursing Standard* 5 (2): 30–32

Illich, I. (1977) *Limits to Medicine.* London: Pelican Books

MacQueen, C.E., Brynes, A.E. and Frost, G.S. (1999) 'Treating obesity: Can the stages of change model help predict outcome measures'. *Journal of Human Nutrition and Dietetics,* 12: 229–236

Naidoo, J. and Wills, J. (2000) *Health Promotion: Foundations for practice* (2nd edn). London: Baillière Tindall

Prochaska, J. and DiClemente, C. (1984) *The Transtheoretical Approach: Crossing traditional foundations of change.* Harnewood: Don Jones/ Irwin

Roden, J. (2004) 'Revisiting the health belief model: Nurses applying it to young families and their health promotion needs'. *Nursing and Health Science,* (6): 1–10

Rosenstock, I. (1966) 'Why people use health services'. *Milbank Memorial Fund Quarterly,* 44: 94–121

Scriven, A. and Orme, J. (2001) *Health Promotion Professional Perspectives* (2nd edn). Basingstoke: Palgrave

Seedhouse, D. (1986) *Health: The foundations for achievement.* Chichester: John Wiley and Sons

Seedhouse, D. (1997) *Health Promotion: Philosophy, prejudice and practice.* Chichester: John Wiley and Sons

Stead, C.K. (ed.) (1977) *The Letters and Journals of Katherine Mansfield: A selection.* London: Allen Lane

Wilson-Barnett, J. and Macleod Clarke, K. (eds) (1993) *Research in Health Promotion and Nursing.* Basingstoke: Macmillan

World Health Organisation (1986) *Ottawa Charter for Health Promotion: An International Conference on Health Promotion,* 17–21 November. Copenhagen: WHO

World Health Organisation (2008) *Closing the Gap in a Generation – Health equity through action on the social determinants of health. Final Report of the Commission on Social Determinants of Health.* Geneva: World Health Organisation

Useful websites

www.engenderhealth.org/res/onc/sti/preventings/sti6p2.html (accessed 5/10/08)

www.nsms.org.uk/public/default.aspx?PageID=10 (accessed 8/10/08)

www.dh.gov.uk/en/Publichealth/Choosinghealth/DH_066342 (accessed 8/10/08)

Chapter 10

Interprofessional Practice and Changing Roles in Nursing

The aim of this chapter is to provide a brief overview regarding interprofessional practice and changes in nurses' roles that have evolved over the past decade. These topics link closely to other chapters, particularly to the provision of health care (Chapter 3).

Outcomes

On completion of this chapter you should be able to:

- understand the concept and context of interprofessional practice;

- appraise the role and function of relevant health and social care professionals;

- appreciate why there has been a need for nurses to change their roles;

- understand the main changes that have occurred to nurses' roles in the past decade.

INTERPROFESSIONAL PRACTICE

The push towards interprofessional collaboration in the field of health care is relatively new and appears to be largely politically driven. As you would expect, since 1948 the provision of health care in the United Kingdom has undergone a variety of changes in terms of organisational restructuring, managerial and economic change. Many of these changes have, unfortunately, often resulted in the fragmentation of health and social care services. This includes those services being managed, at a local level, through different governmental channels, each having very different funding arrangements and dissimilar involvement with independent and voluntary-sector care. In addition to this, professional cultures and forms of accountability within each of the groups have tended to differ significantly.

A perceived solution to this problem by the government has been the attempt, through legislation and initiatives, to develop services at local level that are integrated and that require members of different professions and agencies to work together to develop and improve the provision and delivery of health care services. This principle, despite changes of government, has been central to health and social care provision and delivery policy since the early 1990s. The issues raised in the following commentary will have relevance for wherever you work in the UK.

Definitions

There are a number of terms associated with or used in the context of interprofessional practice. The following are those you are most likely to come into contact with and the definitions are offered in order to clarify their meaning.

- **Uni-disciplinary** – professional groups work independently of one another.
- **Multi-professional/multidisciplinary** – primarily uni-disciplinary – professional groups tend to function independently of one another, but some discussion and negotiation does on occasion occur in order to solve problems outside the scope of the traditional and established professional disciplines.
- **Intra-professional/intra-disciplinary** – a professional group that is further divided into smaller sections, each with its own specific area of specialism like, for example, nursing, – adult, paediatric, mental health, health visiting, district nursing. Intersecting lines of communication and collaboration exist between these professional specialisms.
- **Inter-professional/inter-disciplinary** – intersecting lines of communication and collaboration between different professions and agencies (for example, health and social care, nursing and allied health professionals) are more integrated and all modify their efforts to take account of other team members' contributions. (Clarke, 1991; Funnell, 1995; Leathard, 2003)
- **Collaboration** – can simply mean 'work jointly on an activity or project' (Pearsall, 2001). (Interestingly, the term can also mean 'co-operate traitorously with an enemy'!)

Activity

Consider each of the definitions above and try to relate it to any previous experience you may have had in a care/work environment.

Perceived benefits of interprofessional practice

A review of the literature (Leathard, 1994; Soothill *et al.*, 1995; Barrett, *et al.*, 2005) suggests there is a general consensus, not only in the political arena but also among health and social care professionals, that inter-professional practice can be a positive thing and should provide many benefits to both the practitioners involved and the clients/patients they care for. The identified benefits of such practice include that it:

- allows for streamlining of services (government driven);
- provides for a more effective use of staff;
- offers increased overall quality of service provision;
- provides better use of limited resources.

For the practitioners involved, interprofessional practice also:

- provides a more satisfying work environment;
- can encourage development of mutual respect, mutual cooperation and empathy between professionals;
- should improve communication between different professionals;
- allows all members of the team to understand each other's roles and recognise areas of overlap within the traditional disciplines;
- can encourage a greater understanding of the difference between accountability and responsibility of different team members and what is expected of them.

For service users, benefits include:

- continuity of care;
- consistency of care;
- decrease of ambiguity in the information being given to the patient;
- appropriate referral because of the greater understanding of other professionals' roles;
- care being based on a holistic perspective with the best-placed professionals to meet this agenda.

(Miller *et al.*, 2001)

According to Barrett *et al.* (2005), if such benefits of interprofessional practice are to be maximised, not only will it need to involve complex interactions between practitioners, but also certain other factors and processes will need to be in place. These include:

- knowledge of professional roles;
- willing participation;
- confidence;
- open and honest communication;
- trust and mutual respect;
- shared power;
- support and commitment at a senior level.

Knowledge of professional roles

In order for effective interprofessional practice to take place, it is considered essential that each team member has an understanding of the role and professional boundaries of the other practitioners they may be working with.

Activity

Many of you will already be participating in shared learning with other professional groups – in particular, physiotherapy, occupational therapy and radiography students. It is recommended that you take some time out to talk to them about their specific role and function within the care environment.

Other care professionals that you will be involved with during your training include the following.

District Nurse

A district nurse must be qualified and registered in adult nursing and have undertaken a community specialist practitioner programme (minimum first-degree level). These programmes are normally no less than one academic year (32 weeks) full-time or part-time equivalent (although they may be completed in a shorter period of time where credit is given for prior learning). Community staff nurses can be funded onto the specialist programme via their employing Trust. Alternatively, applicants with the relevant registration and experience can apply for sponsorship via primary care Trusts.

District nurses are an integral part of the primary health care team. They provide nursing care to patients during periods of illness/incapacity in non-hospital settings. This is usually in the patient's own home but can also be in residential care homes, health centres or general practitioner surgeries. Patients may be of any age and include those who are housebound, elderly, terminally ill, disabled and those recently discharged from hospital. The work of district nurses is diverse but their main activities include:

- accepting referrals from other professionals and agencies like, for example, hospitals, general practitioners;
- assessing, planning and managing the care of patients;
- establishing links with patients' families, carers and, where appropriate, working with them to develop their skills in caring for the patient;
- working both intra- and inter-professionally with a range of other professionals and agencies within the NHS, social care, independent and voluntary sector;
- playing a fundamental role in promoting healthy lifestyles and health education/teaching;
- prescribing from an identified list.

www.nhscareers.nhs.uk
www.prospects.ac.uk

Health Visitor

A health visitor must be a qualified and registered nurse, midwife, sick children's nurse or psychiatric nurse with specialist qualifications in community health. Ideally they have had at least two years in practice before undertaking a community specialist public health nursing (health visiting) programme. Most health visitor students are seconded onto a programme by an employer, although a few people may fund themselves.

Health visitors are usually part of the primary health care team and their role involves working with people of all ages in clinics and doctors' surgeries, as well as visiting people in their own homes. Most work, especially with new mothers and children under the age of five, involves advising on such areas as feeding, safety, physical and emotional development and other aspects of health and child care. However, health visitors may also work with people who suffer from chronic illness or live with disability, and marginalised groups such as, for example, the homeless.

The main focus of the work of the health visitor is listening to, advising and supporting individuals and groups, particularly with regard to health promotion and public health, either of which can involve tackling the impact of social inequality on health, and working closely with at-risk or deprived individuals/groups. Activities will vary according to the nature of the individual role, but may include:

- delivering child health programmes and setting up parenting groups;
- identifying the health needs of neighbourhoods and other groups in the community, such as the homeless;
- working with local communities to help them identify and tackle their own health needs and participate in their own health care planning;
- running groups with a specific health aspect like, for example, giving up smoking;
- delivering health improvement programmes that target people with specific needs in such areas as cancer and coronary heart disease;
- working both intra- and inter-professionally with other health and social care practitioners, agencies, independent and voluntary-sector organisations (particularly in relation to child protection).

www.nhscareers.nhs.uk
www.prospects.ac.uk

Social Worker

A qualified social worker will have undertaken a degree or postgraduate qualification approved by the General Social Care Council. Funding for the student to undertake the education/training may come through employer sponsorship, secondment or from the individual.

Social workers practise in a variety of settings, which include service users' homes, schools, hospitals and other public-sector and voluntary organisations. They work with all age groups and support individuals, families and groups in the community within a framework of relevant legislation and procedures, as well as working closely with other organisations including those providing health care. They offer support, advice, counselling and protection to all age groups, although they tend to specialise in one specific area. The main areas in which social workers can specialise are as follows.

Working with children and families
This area can include:

- working to protect children believed to be at risk;

- assisting parents who are experiencing difficulties with bringing up their child/children;
- arranging foster homes or adoption for children who cannot be cared for by their own families;
- helping to keep families together, for example, by giving advice on issues such as drug and alcohol abuse;
- working in children's care homes, and with young offenders in the community.

Working with adults

This area can involve:

- working in a health care setting, assessing the social and emotional needs of patients and their families, helping them adjust to illness;
- evaluating the needs of clients in the community, developing care plans that enable the client to remain living safely and independently at home;
- working with specific groups such as people with HIV or AIDS, the elderly, adults with mental illness, physical disabilities or learning difficulties;
- working to protect vulnerable adults.

Work with offenders

In Northern Ireland, Wales and Scotland, social workers can choose to specialise in working with offenders. Activities again will vary according to the specialist area but can include:

- conducting interviews with service users and their families to assess and review the situation;
- organising and managing packages of support for users of the service, recommending and sometimes making decisions about the best course of action for the service user;
- working interprofessionally with health care professionals, other agencies, the independent and voluntary sectors;
- giving evidence in court.

www.gscc.org.uk
www.learndirect-advice.co.uk

Willing participation

According to Hennemann *et al.* (1995) and Molyneux (2001), high levels of motivation and the willingness of the participants is key to the effectiveness of any interprofessional collaboration. Maintaining such motivation and willingness, even if unsatisfactory experiences of inter-professional practice are encountered, is obviously very important.

Confidence

Writers such as Leathard (2003) suggest that the most basic requirement for interprofessional collaboration must be the individual's own professional competence. They argue that until the practitioner feels confident that they are expert in their own field, and are so regarded by their peers, they are unlikely to feel sufficiently secure to fully engage in 'sharing' practice with others outside their own professional arena. Personal levels of confidence within the practice area will increase as you progress through your student nurse programme and will continue to do so after you qualify.

Open and honest communication

According to Barrett *et al.* (2005), open and honest communication is linked very closely to internal feelings associated again with an individual's level of confidence. It also involves, suggest Hornby and Atkins (2000), the need for the participants to set aside any preconceived ideas and judgements they may have about other professions involved in the collaborative practice.

Trust and mutual respect

Stapleton (1998, p. 14) views trust as 'an essential attribute of collaboration', and considers it as another element that develops over time through repeated positive interprofessional experiences, both in the classroom and in practice. Mutual respect, according to Barrett *et al.* (2005), develops when, again, all participants feel valued through explicit acknowledgement of each profession's unique contribution to the overall process.

Shared power

Stapleton (1998) identifies shared power as being based on non-hierarchical relationships. However, historically, power tends to be located within the medical profession. Although this does seem to be changing slowly, there still appears to be some way to go before they relinquish their traditionally held power base in favour of a true non-hierarchical relationship with other health and social care professionals (particularly to the so-called 'semi-professionals' such as nursing and social work).

Support and commitment at a senior level

According to Fieldgrass (1992, cited in Barrett *et al.*, 2005), commitment to interprofessional working must also occur at a senior level as collaborative practice can be expensive in terms of time and resources. If such practice is imposed from senior level then support for the professionals involved in its development must also come from that level. This, according to Barrett *et al.*, (2005), needs to involve such strategies as encouraging reflection through clinical supervision, education and training, team development and establishing the guidelines relating to the parameters within which individual professions work.

POSTSCRIPT AND A NOTE OF CAUTION

Despite the recognised benefits there are still some difficulties or barriers to effective and widespread interprofessional practice. These include:

- **organisational issues** – (between health and social services, such as, for example, disparity of boundaries and centres of control);
- **operational matters** – different budgetary and planning sequences and procedures;
- **monetary factors** – including different funding structures and sources of financial resources;
- **status and validity** – social care is directed through democratically elected and appointed agencies, i.e. local authorities, whereas health care is directed by policy from central government through the NHS;
- **professional issues** are numerous and include:
  - problems associated with differing ideologies, values and language;
  - conflicting views about users;
  - separate training backgrounds;
  - differing organisational boundaries and professional loyalties;
  - inequalities in status and pay;
  - lack of clarity about roles and historical prejudices;
  - professional defence of professions and an unwillingness to dilute them in any way (professional protectionism);
  - differences between specialisms, expertise and skills – this can include medical practitioners (and unfortunately can occur intra-professionally as well as inter-professionally).

(Leathard, 2003; Pietroni, 1992)

However, ongoing government policy legislation and directives and the inclusion of interprofessional education and training for health and social care professionals seek to lessen the impact of the above factors.

Further reading

For a range of issues associated with interprofessional practice you can visit **www.practicebasedlearning.org;** click on 'resources' and follow the links for interprofessional learning in practice.

CHANGING ROLES IN NURSING

Why the need for change?

The International Council of Nurses (**www.icn.ch/definition.htm**) offers a definition of nursing that encompasses the vast arena of care that nurses deliver. While it is accepted that not all nurses are involved in all the aspects of nursing described at any one time, nurses still need to be flexible, adaptable and innovative to be able to respond to the changing needs and perceptions of their patients and clients. In addition, a market-driven health service and ever-changing reforms require the nursing role to be continuously evolving and changing.

The ICN definition of nursing

Nursing encompasses autonomous and collaborative care of individuals of all ages, families, groups and communities, sick or well and in all settings. Nursing includes the promotion of health, prevention of illness, and the care of ill, disabled and dying people. Advocacy, promotion of a safe environment, research, participation in shaping health policy and in-patient and health systems management, and education are also key nursing roles.

The NHS Plan

Probably the most profound impact on a nurse's work life in recent years has been the introduction of *The NHS Plan* (Department of Health, 2000). This has been the biggest change to health care in England since the NHS was formed in 1948, and *The Plan* sets out how increased funding and reform aim to redress geographical inequalities, improve service standards and extend patient choice. It also outlines a new delivery system for the NHS, changes for social services and changes for NHS staff groups. Indeed, one section of *The Plan* actually states that it 'encourages nurses and other staff to extend their roles'.

Many of the changes in the health service today, which include the role of the nurse, have been driven by patients – indeed, they were major contributors to *The NHS Plan*. Patient and client perceptions and expectations of their health care have risen as information on medical and nursing roles has been made more accessible and transparent. However, the changing roles of other health care professionals have also had an impact on the nurse's role and, in some instances, have lead to the creation of completely new roles for nurses.

Changing policy, changing practice (NMC, 2005a)

The NMC has summarised the changes in the registered nurse's role over the past decades (see below). Although currently a student, you need to have an awareness of changes in the role you will assume once registered, and an understanding of your future professional body's viewpoint on this:

> The practice of nurses, midwives and health visitors is constantly evolving and changing. Nurses, midwives and health visitors have continually adjusted the scope of their practice to meet changing health needs. Changes in health policy, such as the shift towards a primary care led NHS, an increasing emphasis on public health and community based services, together with technological advances and developments in scientific knowledge have required all the health care professions to develop in new ways. These changes have increased the skills and decision-making required of all nurses, midwives and health visitors. What was once unthinkable – nurses carrying out endoscopies, acting as specialists in diverse areas of care such as diabetes and behavioural therapy, working as first assistant to surgeons, and running their own clinics in acute and primary care; midwives developing and leading total programmes of care for pregnant women with severe social and/or emotional difficulties,

directing the development of clinical guidelines, and specialising in supporting women and their partners following early pregnancy loss; health visitors co-ordinating community development work, specialising in child protection, and leading multi-agency work on service development for older people – is now becoming commonplace. *The scope of professional practice* encouraged nurses, midwives and health visitors to take on new roles and activities to adapt to meet changing health care needs. There are few tasks which nurses, midwives and health visitors cannot undertake legally and many former 'extended role' activities, e.g. intravenous drug administration, cannulation, venepuncture and ECGs, now form the expected skill base of all registered practitioners.

The clinical nurse specialist role in areas such as infection control, tissue viability, stoma care, continence and so on has existed informally since the 1970s. Clinical nurse specialists were seen as experts in a particular area of care or with a particular client group, with post-qualification education and a research base firmly grounded in nursing. The title was not regulated and post-holders usually achieved such jobs through extensive experience and appropriate post-registration courses. Clinical nurse specialists were usually managed within the nursing service. Nurse practitioners developed first in primary care in the late 1980s and offered an alternative service to that provided by general practitioners or filled gaps in service provision such as providing primary care to homeless people. Nurse practitioners diagnose, refer, prescribe and provide complete episodes of care for clients with undifferentiated health problems. In the 1990s, posts emerged in secondary care with the titles of nurse practitioner, advanced practitioner and advanced nurse practitioner. Such posts frequently involve nurses giving care or performing tasks previously done by doctors. For example, in some trusts advanced neo-natal practitioners are replacing junior doctors on the senior house officer rota in special care baby units; surgical nurse practitioners run pre-admission clinics, clerk patients and organise theatre lists, other nurse practitioners work across the primary/secondary care interface and prescribe within protocols for conditions such as hypertension, asthma and so on.

Latterly, consultant nurse, midwife and health visitor posts have been introduced in the NHS. Consultant nurses, midwives and health visitors are expected to be competent to initiate and lead significant practice, education and service development.

Four key areas of responsibility have been defined – expert practice; professional leadership and consultancy; education and development; and practice and service development linked to research and evaluation.

Consultant nurses, midwives and health visitors are to have been educated to masters or doctorate level, be registered as a nurse, midwife or health visitor, and hold additional professional qualifications. The development of such posts has been described as a national priority and it has been suggested that these posts should be used to tackle particular service problems and lead service development in government determined priority areas.

In the past, registration was seen as a licence to practise for life. In today's world however the importance of all practitioners ensuring that their skills and expertise remain relevant to the needs of their patients and clients and constantly learning and updating their knowledge and skills is increasingly recognised.

In light of the increasing speed and nature of change in the professional practice of many nurses, midwives and health visitors outlined above, the NMC recognised and responded to the need to consider how its regulatory frameworks protected the public.

(NMC, 2005a)

Activity

Having read the NMC statement above, list any specialist roles you have seen undertaken by nurses in your placement areas.

New nursing roles

One of the reasons nurses are changing their roles is that the organisations within health care have also changed their roles, or at least have had to change the way they work, in order to accommodate new technologies, new legislation (both UK and European) and new government initiatives. Some of the new roles nurses are now undertaking are considered below. This is not an exhaustive list, but highlights the concept of nurses working beyond their initial registration.

Nurse consultants and midwife consultants

Nurse consultants and midwife consultant posts were first established in 1999. They are central to the process of health service modernisation, helping to provide patients with services that are fast and convenient. Nurse consultants and midwife consultants are experienced registered nurses and midwives, who will specialise in a particular field of health care. All nurse and midwife consultants spend a minimum of 50 per cent of their time working directly with patients, ensuring that people using the NHS continue to benefit from the very best nursing and midwifery skills. In addition, the nurse consultants are responsible for developing personal practice, being involved in research and evaluation and contributing to education, training and development.

Each consultant role will be very different, depending upon the needs of the employer, but nurses and midwives working at this level are among the highest paid of their professions (**www.nhscareers.nhs.uk**).

Advanced Nurse Practitioner

Publication of the document *Making a Difference – Strengthening the nursing, midwifery and health visiting contribution to health and health care* (Department of Health, 1999a) outlined a new career framework for nurses. This framework includes the development of advanced nursing posts that are intended to extend the career opportunities for expert nurses who wish to remain in clinically focused roles.

The advanced nurse practitioner is one of these posts, and can be found in both primary and secondary care settings. The NMC (2005b p. 2) define the role thus:

> Advanced nurse practitioners are highly experienced and educated members of the care team who are able to diagnose and treat [your] healthcare needs and refer [you] to an appropriate specialist if required.

The Royal College of Nursing (2008) further defines an advanced nurse practitioner as:

> A registered nurse who has undertaken a specific course of study of at least first degree (honours) level and who:
>
> * makes professional autonomous decisions, for which he or she is accountable;

- receives patients with undifferentiated and undiagnosed problems and makes an assessment of their health care needs, based on highly developed nursing knowledge and skills, including skills not usually exercised by nurses, such as physical examination;
- screens patients for disease risk factors and early signs of illness;
- makes a differential diagnosis using decision-making and problem-solving skills;
- develops with the patient an ongoing nursing care plan for health, with an emphasis on preventative measures;
- orders necessary investigations, and provides treatment and care both individually, as part of a team, and through referral to other agencies;
- has a supportive role in helping people to manage and live with illness;
- provides counselling and health education;
- has the authority to admit or discharge patients from their caseload, and refer patients to other health care providers as appropriate;
- works collaboratively with other health care professionals and disciplines;
- provides a leadership and consultancy function as required.

Nurse prescriber

Since 1994 some nurses have been able to prescribe medicines for certain groups of patients. In 1999 the *Review of Prescribing, Supply and Administration* (Department of Health, 1999b) put forward key principles for the extension of prescribing rights. These principles included the need for appropriate training, regulation and updating, and the need for prescribing to take place within a framework of accountability and competency. In 2007 the NMC further clarified who could prescribe what, and what qualifications were required:

> **Qualified Nurse Prescribers** (NMC, 2007, Standard 1)
> Any qualified and registered independent prescriber may prescribe all Prescription Only Medicines for all medical conditions.

In addition, nurse independent prescribers may also prescribe some controlled drugs.

The Medicinal Products: Prescription by Nurses Act 1992 and subsequent amendments allow nurses who have recorded their qualification on the NMC register to become nurse prescribers. There are differing levels of prescribers.

- **Community practitioner nurse prescribers:** those who have successfully undertaken a programme of preparation to prescribe from the community practitioner nurse prescribers' formulary.
- **Independent/supplementary nurse prescriber:** those trained to make a diagnosis and prescribe the appropriate treatment – they may also, in cases where a doctor has made an initial diagnosis, go on to prescribe or review medication and change the drug, dosage, timing, frequency or route of administration of any medication as part of a clinical management plan (a tripartite arrangement with a doctor or dentist, the patient and the supplementary prescriber).
- **Nurse independent prescribers:** can prescribe all Prescription Only Medicines (including some controlled drugs) and all medication that can be supplied by a pharmacist or bought over the counter; however, they must only prescribe drugs that are within their area of expertise and competence.

Further information

If you wish to know more about nurse prescribing, access the NMC website at **www.nmc-uk.org** and read the position statement.

Modern Matron (from: *Modern Matrons – Improving the patient experience*, Department of Health, 2003)

In 2001, as part of the *NHS Plan*, the NHS re-introduced the role of matron, a role that had disappeared in the late 1960s, but this time in a modern and far more important role.

Modern Matrons were introduced to provide strong leadership on wards and to be highly visible and accessible to patients. They lead by example in driving up standards of clinical care and empower nurses to take on a greater range of clinical tasks to help improve patient care. Also, crucially, they have the power to get the basics right for patients – clean wards, good food, quality care.

The new matron role positions nursing at the very heart of the NHS modernisation process. It is part of a profound cultural change that puts the patient first. In such a system, effective frontline leaders are vitally important in achieving delivery. The ten key responsibilities of matrons are:

- leading by example;
- making sure patients get quality care;

- ensuring staffing is appropriate to patient needs;
- empowering nurses to take on a wider range of clinical tasks;
- improving hospital cleanliness;
- ensuring patients' nutritional needs are met;
- improving wards for patients;
- making sure patients are treated with respect;
- preventing hospital-acquired infection;
- resolving problems for patients and their relatives by building closer relationships.

Assistant Practitioner

In addition to enhancing the role of registered nurses, a new grade of Assistant Practitioner has been introduced under the Skills for Health Framework, this role being relevant to all health and social care professions and not just nursing.

Skills for Health, established in April 2002, is part of the NHS and covers the whole health sector – NHS, independent and voluntary employers. One of its remits was to develop a career framework for all personnel working within health care. The Assistant Practitioner is one such role and involves delivering protocol-based clinical care, which had previously been in the remit of registered professionals, under the direction and supervision of a registered practitioner. As you can see from the chart below, the assistant practitioner is at level 4.

Key Elements of the Career Framework
(**www.skillsforhealth.org.uk**)

More Senior Staff – Level 9
Staff with the ultimate responsibility for clinical caseload decision-making and full on-call accountability.

Consultant Practitioners – Level 8
Staff working at a very high level of clinical expertise and/or who have responsibility for planning of services.

Advanced Practitioners – Level 7
Experienced clinical professionals who have developed their skills and theoretical knowledge to a very high standard. They are empowered to make high-level clinical decisions and will often have their own caseload. Non-clinical staff at Level 7 will typically be managing a number of service areas.

Senior Practitioners/Specialist Practitioners – Level 6
Staff who would have a higher degree of autonomy and responsibility than 'practitioners' in the clinical environment, or who would be managing one or more service areas in the non-clinical environment.

Practitioners – Level 5
Most frequently registered practitioners in their first and second post-registration/professional qualification jobs.

Assistant Practitioners/Associate Practitioners – Level 4
Probably studying for a foundation degree, BTEC higher or HND. Some of their remit will involve them in delivering protocol-based clinical care that had previously been in the remit of registered professionals, under the direction and supervision of a state-registered practitioner.

Senior Healthcare Assistants/Technicians – Level 3
Have a higher level of responsibility than support workers, probably studying for, or have attained NVQ level 3, or Assessment of Prior Experiential Learning (APEL).

Support Workers – Level 2
Frequently with the job title of 'Healthcare Assistant' or 'Healthcare Technician' – probably studying for or have attained NVQ Level 2.

Initial Entry Level Jobs – Level 1
Such as 'domestics' or 'cadets', requiring very little formal education or previous knowledge, skills or experience in delivering, or supporting, the delivery of health care.

For further information about Skills for Health and its role, visit its website at **www.skillsforhealth.org.uk**

REFERENCES

Barrett, G., Sellman, D. and Thomas, J. (2005) *Multi-disciplinary Working in Health Care and Social Care – Professional perspectives*. Hampshire: Palgrave Macmillan

Clarke, P. (1991) 'Towards a conceptual framework for developing interdisciplinary teams in gerontology: Cognitive and ethical'. *Gerontology and Geriatrics Education*, 12 (1): 79–96

Department of Health (1999a) *Making a Difference – Strengthening the nursing, midwifery and health visiting contribution to health and health care*. London: Department of Health

Department of Health (1999b) *Review of Prescribing, Supply and Administration of Medicines*. London: Department of Health

Department of Health (2000) *The NHS Plan*. London: Department of Health

Department of Health (2003) *Modern Matrons – Improving the patient experience*. London: Department of Health

Funnell, P. (1995) 'Exploring the value of interprofessional shared learning', cited in Soothill, K., Mackay, L. and Webb, C. *Interprofessional Relations in Health Care* (pp. 163–171). London: Edward Arnold

Henneman, E., Lee, J. and Cohen, J. (1995) 'A concept analysis of collaboration'. *Journal of Advanced Nursing* (21): 103–9

Hornby, S. and Atkins, J. (2000) *Collaborative Care: Multi-disciplinary, interagency and interpersonal* (2nd edn). Oxford: Blackwell Science

Leathard, A. (1994) *Going Multi-disciplinary. Working together for health and welfare*. London: Routledge

Leathard, A. (2003) *Interprofessional Collaboration: From policy to practice in health and social care*. Hove: Brunner-Routledge

Miller, C., Freeman, M. and Ross, N. (2001) *Interprofessional Practice in Health and Social Care: Challenging the shared learning agenda*. London: Arnold

Molyneux, J. (2001) 'Multi-disciplinary teamworking: what makes teams work well?', *Journal of Multi-disciplinary Care* 15: 29–35

Nursing and Midwifery Council (2005a) *Changing Policy, Changing Practice*. London: NMC

Nursing and Midwifery Council (2005b) *Implementation of a framework for the standard of post-registration nursing*. London: NMC

Nursing and Midwifery Council (2007) *Standards for Medicines Management*. London: NMC

Pearsall, J. (2001) (ed.) *The Concise Oxford Dictionary* (10th edn revised). London: Oxford University Press

Pietroni, P. (1992) 'Towards reflective practice – the languages of health and social care'. *Journal of Interprofessional Care* (1) Spring: 7–16

Royal College of Nursing (2008) *Advanced Nurse Practitioners – An RCN guide to the advanced nurse practitioner role, competencies and programme accreditation*. London: RCN

Soothill, K., Mackay, L. and Webb, C. (1995) *Multi-disciplinary Relations in Health Care*. London: Edward Arnold

Stapleton, S.R. (1998) 'Team-building: making collaborative practice work'. *Journal of Midwifery*, 43: 12–18

Useful websites

www.dh.gov.uk (accessed 15/10/08)

www.icn.ch/definition.htm (accessed 16/10/08)

www.nhscareers.nhs.uk (accessed 15/10/08)

www.nmc-uk.org (accessed 16/10/08)

www.skillsforhealth.org.uk/careerframework/key_elements.php (accessed 15/10/08)

www.nhscareers.nhs.uk/nhs-knowledge_base/data/7806.html (accessed 15/10/08)

www.nhscareers.nhs.uk/nhs-knowledge_base/data/5632.html (accessed 15/10/08)

www.learndirect-advice.co.uk/helpwithyourcareer/jobprofiles/profiles/profile709 (accessed 15/10/08)

www.gscc.org.uk/Training+and+learning/Become+a+social+worker/Becoming+a+social+worker+FAQs (accessed 15/10/08)

www.prospects.ac.uk/cms/ShowPage/Home_page/Explore_types_of_jobs/Type (accessed 15/10/08)

Chapter 11

Reflection and Professional Development

This chapter looks at reflection and two aspects of professional development: clinical supervision and portfolios. Reflection surrounds both these professional development aspects and, although it is a duty of a registered nurse to undertake professional development, you will be introduced to the concept within your training. It will give you an insight into how reflective skills gained as a student are carried on into registered nurse practice.

Outcomes

On completion of this chapter you should be able to:

- understand the concept of reflection as a learning strategy;

- describe the process of reflection and exercise the skills required to carry this out;

- discuss the advantages of using reflection in practice;

- have an understanding of the need to maintain a portfolio;

- appreciate the NMC's position on personal professional profiles;

- consider how you might structure your own portfolio;

- appreciate the concept and advantages of clinical supervision.

REFLECTION

Reflection is associated with learning from experience and is viewed as an important strategy for nurses, who should embrace lifelong learning. The term 'reflection' is often used synonymously with the terms 'reflective practice' and 'reflective learning', and literature around the subject indicates that most agree that it is an active, conscious process where an experience is explored in order to gain new understandings and to learn something new. Dewey stated this as far back as 1938 when he simply said: 'we learn by doing and realising what we did' (Dewey, 1938, cited in Jasper, 2006). Moon (2004) agrees with this when stating that reflective learning is where the learner considers their practice honestly and critically and is often initiated when the individual practitioner encounters some problematic aspect of practice and attempts to make sense of it. However, Jasper (2006, p. 44) makes the distinction between reflection and reflective practice: 'using reflection alone in order to learn is not reflective practice . . . practice is about doing something. Therefore reflective practice means using the reflective process to inform practice in some way'.

Jasper (2006) also points out that reflection is a learning strategy that can be achieved either formally or informally and can be outside the formal learning environment. It can help bridge the theory–practice gap that students often find so challenging: as a student you develop skills for learning in an educational setting – analysing literature, writing essays, etc. – while, in practice, you learn from the clinical setting – working with your mentor and other health care professionals, performing new skills, assessing patients' needs, planning their care, etc. Reflection can help to integrate these learning processes by using the theory gained from the educational setting to inform everyday working practices.

There are many different models for reflection, with no one being better than any other – it is a matter of personal choice which is used, but the consensus from nursing literature is that reflection should be structured to enable learning to come as a result. Price (2002) suggests that reflection is more comfortable and effective if a step-by-step approach is used, and most of the reflective models acknowledge this with a broad outline of the stages being:

- thinking back over a situation;
- possibly discussing the incident with other people;
- re-evaluating the experience to seek possible new understandings;
- checking out new knowledge;
- developing an action plan for the future.

(Whitehead and Mason, 2003)

Good reflective practice underpins good professional practice in that reflection enables practitioners to review their progress and identify areas which have been successfully developed, and those which are in need of further development. It enhances a commitment to 'lifelong learning' and continuous professional development (Somerset Academy, 2005).

MODELS OF REFLECTION

As mentioned above, there are many models of reflection to choose from. Outlined below are three of the most widely used.

Gibbs' (1998) reflective cycle

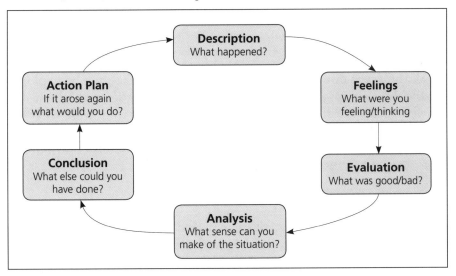

Figure 1 Gibbs' (1998) reflective cycle

Gibbs' (1998) reflective cycle (see Figure 1) is fairly straightforward and encourages a clear description of the situation, analysis of feelings, evaluation of the experience, analysis to make sense of the experience, conclusion where other options are considered, and reflection upon experience to examine what you would do if the situation arose again. Jasper (2003) outlines the stages of Gibbs' cycle in greater detail and gives suggestions on how it should be used.

Stage 1: Description of the event

Describe in detail the event you are reflecting on. Include, for example: where were you; who else was there; why were you there; what were you doing; what were other people doing; what was the context of the event; what happened; what was your part in this; what parts did the other people play; what was the result?

Stage 2: Feelings

At this stage try to recall and explore the things that were going on inside your head, i.e. why does this event stick in your mind? Include, for example: how were you feeling when the event started; what were you thinking about at the time; how did it make you feel; how did other people make you feel; how did you feel about the outcome of the event; what do you think about it now?

Stage 3: Evaluation

Try to evaluate or make a judgement about what has happened. Consider what was good about the experience and what was bad about the experience or didn't go so well.

Stage 4: Analysis

Break the event down into its component parts so they can be explored separately. You may need to ask more detailed questions about the answers to the last stage. Include, for example: what went well; what did you do well; what did others do well; what went wrong or did not turn out as it should have done; in what way did you or others contribute to this?

Stage 5: Conclusion

This differs from the evaluation stage in that now you have explored the issue from different angles and have a lot of information on which to base your judgement. It is here that you are likely to develop insight into your own and other people's behaviour in terms of how they contributed to the outcome of the event. Remember that the purpose of reflection is to learn from an experience. Without detailed analysis and honest exploration that occurs during all the previous stages, it is unlikely that all aspects of the event will be taken into account, and therefore valuable opportunities for learning can be missed. During this stage you should ask yourself what you could have done differently.

Stage 6: Action plan

During this stage you should think yourself forward into encountering the event again and plan what you would do – would you act differently or would you be likely to do the same?

Here the cycle is tentatively completed and suggests that, should the event occur again, it will be the focus of another reflective cycle.

Johns' (2002) model for structured reflection: Version 13

Johns' (2002) model for structured reflection can be used as a guide for analysis of a critical incident or for general reflection on experience, and is useful for more complex analyses. Johns believes that the reflector should work with a supervisor as he considers that through sharing reflections greater understanding of those experiences can be achieved, rather than the reflector undertaking a lone exercise. The stages of Johns' (2002) model of structured reflection are:

- what issues seem significant to pay attention to?
- how was I feeling and what made me feel that way?
- what was I trying to achieve?
- did I respond effectively and in tune with my values?
- what were the consequences of my action on the patient, others and myself?
- how were others feeling?
- what made them feel that way?
- what factors influenced the way I was feeling, thinking or responding?
- what knowledge did or might have informed me?
- to what extent did I act for the best?
- how does this situation connect with my previous experience?
- how might I respond more effectively given this situation again?
- what would be the consequences of alternative actions for the patient, others and myself?
- how do I now feel about this experience?
- am I more able to support myself and others better as a consequence?
- am I more available to work with patients, families and staff to help them meet their needs?

Stephenson's reflective model (1993)

Another very useful framework was developed by a nursing student (Stephenson, 1993, cited in Palmer *et al.*, 1994) as a result of four years' experience of reflecting on her practice. This framework takes a critical approach, moving from personal reflection to consideration of ethical, political and social issues. Essentially, Stephenson's framework involves considering:

- what was my role in this situation?
- did I feel comfortable or uncomfortable – why?
- what actions did I take?

- how did I and others act?
- was it appropriate?
- how could I have improved the situation for myself, the patient, my mentor?
- what can I achieve in the future?
- do I feel as if I have learnt anything new about myself?
- did I expect anything different to happen – what and why?
- has it changed my way of thinking in any way?
- what knowledge from theory and research can I apply to this situation?
- what broader issues, for example ethical, political or social, arise from this situation?
- what do I think about these broader issues?

(Stephenson, 1993, cited in Palmer *et al.*, 1994, pp. 56–57)

Using reflective frameworks

Regardless of whichever model for reflection is used, Price (2002) suggests that the challenge of using reflective frameworks is often in ensuring that you have considered the following:

- did you consider your own prejudices?
- did you avoid seeing only the familiar and/or one perspective?
- did you consider what others might have intended to signal through their behaviour?
- did you make use of and check out all the available information?
- did you actually learn something new?
- did you form an action plan of how to approach this differently in future?

The benefits of practising reflectively

Jasper (2006, p. 53) lists who she believes benefits from nurses practising reflectively. They are:

- the individual, in terms of providing individualised care, identifying their learning needs, and learning from experience;
- the patient, in terms of higher quality and standards of care, and care designed to meet their own unique needs;
- the employer, in terms of standards of care achieved, in having a continually developing workforce which recognises its own professional development;

- the profession, in terms of self-regulation of the practitioners, in developing the nursing knowledge base, in contributing to increasing the status of nursing and recognition of nurses' contribution to patient care.

Activity

To see if Gibbs' reflective cycle can help you reflect on aspects of your practice, recall a recent clinical nursing situation in which you were involved. Write your description of the situation, and then apply the rest of Gibbs' model to reflect on the situation.

Reflective writing – Keeping a journal/reflective diary

The purpose of reflective writing is to support the process of reflection while, at the same time, providing evidence of learning (Hurford, 2009). Many people find it takes time to develop reflective skills, so it is important to build on this early in your course (Cottrell, 2003). Reflective writing requires a commitment of time and energy as it involves looking at a situation in depth, but it is an excellent basis for professional development, both as a student and when you become a registered nurse. The reasons why writing, rather than thinking or verbalising, are beneficial are listed as follows.

Writing:

- is an active process;
- organises and encourages deep thoughts and feelings;
- enables the gaining of more control over thoughts, emotions, responses and behaviour;
- encourages self-awareness, self-diagnosis and honesty;
- encourages examination of the negative, development of the positive and can reveal uncertainties which need exploring;
- is done for the purpose of learning;
- provides a way of exploring a range of issues from different perspectives;
- stimulates change.

(Jasper, 2006; Kitson, 2005; Cottrell, 2003)

Records of reflection over time should be kept in a portfolio as evidence of professional development and contribute to your personal development plan. This is essential for registered nurses, but is also expected of, and is good practice for students. It allows you to look for themes that reoccur and perhaps are not resolved, or conflicts that present themselves in a variety of forms. It also provides a safe base for you to explore your feelings, which can be challenging as you may discover truths about yourself that are embarrassing or make you feel uncomfortable. For this reason, Burns and Bulman (2000) suggest journals should be kept private and only selected aspects made available for more public reading.

Any of the frameworks mentioned already in this chapter can be used to write reflectively or, if you prefer, you can write using 'free-flowing' text. As you become used to this process you will develop confidence in your own evaluation and judgement of your work. The important aspect is that you are writing about your experiences, therefore you should write in the first person. Focus on yourself and avoid using reflection as a way of blaming or taking out anger on others. It is your own role you need to consider and how you would make a similar situation more manageable next time. Openness, honesty and critical analysis are the key features you need to consider, along with identification of any actions required in terms of your development.

Reflection is not all about 'clinical incidents'. You can reflect on your course by focusing on your development and progress as a whole, both academically and clinically. Cottrell (2008) suggests you consider:

- your feelings about your course, the lecturers, other students, your progress;
- things you find difficult – challenges;
- changes in your attitude or motivation;
- how you tackle tasks – your strategies;
- things you find out about yourself;
- thoughts about how you learn best;
- ideas that arise from your studies;
- how different areas of studies link up;
- how your studies relate to real life.

These aspects can act as a basis for discussion with your tutors, along with any possible options you may have to address any issues arising from your reflection.

Activity

Using a different model from that of Gibbs, write a short reflective account of a recent situation you encountered while studying at university (not a clinical event). Compare the reflective model used with Gibbs' model and consider which one you found the most useful.

PROFESSIONAL DEVELOPMENT

The following topics – portfolios and profiles and clinical supervision – give a brief outline of what is expected of you when you register as a nurse with the NMC. They both involve reflection and are therefore discussed briefly in the following pages.

Portfolios and profiles

The demonstration of professional competence is a crucial element of being a registered, accountable practitioner (Jasper, 2006). The NMC states that all registered nurses in the UK are required to create and maintain a portfolio and, within that, a personal professional profile demonstrating fitness to remain eligible to practice. It should outline your career progress and identify learning opportunities for the future.

You may or may not be familiar with the concept of maintaining your own portfolio but, on the whole, any portfolio you may be required to compile as a student will ask you to evidence pre-specified criteria (achievement of competences and learning outcomes, etc.). Post-registration portfolios have a different focus as they require evidence to demonstrate fitness for continuing practice. However, there is sometimes confusion as to what a profile is and what a portfolio is, so Brown (1995) offers the following definitions:

Portfolio

'A private collection of evidence which demonstrates the continuing acquisition of skills, knowledge, attitudes, understanding and achievements. It is both retrospective and prospective, as well as reflecting the current stage of development and activity of the individual' (Brown, 1995, p. 3).

Profile

A collection of evidence which is selected from your portfolio for a particular purpose, and for the attention of a particular audience. Therefore an array of profiles can be developed to meet different needs, for example when applying for a job, for professional development review, etc.

Jasper (2006, p.155) suggests that Brown's definitions emphasise several features.

- Their individual nature – portfolios are unique to the person compiling them and provide a permanent record of that person's professional history.
- They are 'dynamic' in nature in that they reflect the past but anticipate and plan for the future.
- They document and record specific 'attributes' of the individual concerned.
- They comprise various types of 'evidence'.

The NMC states that a profile is:

> a record of career progress and professional development. It is not a CV, a daily diary of events or your whole life history! A profile is a flexible but comprehensive account of your professional development. However, it is more than a record of achievement. It is based on a regular process of reflection and recording what you learn from everyday experiences, as well as planned learning activity. Your profile is your personal document. It does not belong to the NMC or your employer and its contents are private and confidential to you.
>
> **www.nmc-uk.org**

Jasper (2006) highlights the benefits of maintaining a portfolio as helping you to:

- assess your current standards of practice;
- develop your analytical skills through reflection on what you do;
- review and evaluate past experience and learning to help you plan for the future;
- provide effective and current information if you apply for a job or a course;
- demonstrate experiential learning which may allow you to obtain credit towards further qualifications.

Organising and documenting your information (NMC, 2008a)

There is no approved format for a profile. Whatever format you choose – ring binder, box file, disk or one of the profiles available commercially – the main factors should be flexibility, accessibility and confidentiality. You should be aware that your profile will contain personal information, so it should not be accessible to others without your permission. At the same time, you should not document any information that could identify patients, clients or carers as this could constitute a breach of confidentiality. For these reasons, you could consider dividing your profile into two sections: one containing confidential information (i.e. reflections, etc.) and the other containing material that the NMC may require for audit purposes – see the NMC *Prep Handbook* (2008a) regarding audit.

As there is no definite format as to what should be included in a portfolio, because it is personal to you, you might wish to consider some suggestions:

- personal details – CV and employment record;
- educational and academic record;
- personal and professional development (past and present);
- professional work with key learning points;
- reflective reviews with key learning points and an action plan;
- critical incident analysis;
- copies of articles written or other written publications;
- non-nursing experiences;
- future development and career aspirations.

Boud *et al.* (1985) give guidelines or tips on how to develop and maintain a portfolio that may be of help.

- Seek out a method that suits you – it is important to keep your portfolio personal – write about what it is important for you, not what others say you should.
- Be frank, honest and spontaneous in your entries – use your own words, say what you feel.
- Have a positive approach when writing – write regularly and stick at it.
- Feel free to express yourself in diagrams, pictures or other types of material.
- A portfolio is meant to be a workbook – work through entries a number of times, go back to early entries and further reflect on them.
- Focus on things that are important – do not waste time on trivialities.

- Do not be rigid in the way you keep your portfolio – be prepared to change your methods.
- Record experiences as soon as possible after they happen, and in as much detail as possible.
- Important issues may need to be shared with others, and record your feedback – this will deepen your understanding of situations.

(adapted from Boud *et al.*, 1985)

Clinical supervision

Clinical supervision is a term that has been used by registered nurses and other health care professionals to provide a purposeful, practice-focused relationship that enables the nurse to reflect on their practice with the support of a skilled supervisor (Peate, 2006). It was introduced in the workplace for nurses during the 1990s, following the Department of Health's document *Vision for the Future* (Department of Health, 1993), as a way of using reflective practice and shared experiences as part of continuing professional development (CPD). The concept, however, has been long established in professions such as midwifery, social work, psychotherapy and counselling.

The Department of Health (1993, p. 3) defines clinical supervision as:

> a formal process of professional support and learning which enables individual practitioners to develop knowledge and competence, assume responsibility for their own practice and enhance consumer protection and safety in care in complex clinical situations.

Clinical supervision also has the support of the NMC (2008b) and RCN (2002), who state that it enables registered nurses to:

- reflect on nursing practice;
- identify solutions to problems;
- increase understanding of professional issues;
- improve standards of patient care;
- further develop their skills and knowledge;
- enhance understanding of their own practice;
- identify room for improvement;
- devise new ways of learning;
- gain professional support.

Clinical supervision is different from any discussion you may have with your line manager when you are registered in that it involves stepping back and reflecting on practice with a clinical supervisor who is external to your immediate workplace. It should not be confused with appraisal, development review or any other management activity. It is not currently a mandatory requirement from the NMC, and anything said in sessions should be confidential.

The clinical supervision sessions themselves will be carefully structured and managed with clearly defined aims and objectives. Ground rules and responsibilities will be clearly defined and there should be a contract of commitment from both supervisor and supervisees in order for it to be a meaningful exercise.

There are various models or approaches to clinical supervision; one-to-one supervision, group supervision, or peer group supervision. The choice of approach will depend upon a number of factors, including personal choice, access to supervision, length of experience, qualifications, availability of supervisory groups, etc. However, all partaking in clinical supervision will have a supervisor who is a skilled professional and assists other practitioners in the development of their skills, knowledge and professional values. Fitzgerald (2000, p. 155) believes that:

> within these types of supervisory relationships reflection plays an important role in the clinical supervision process. The use of a reflective framework facilitates a structured approach to the agenda of the supervisory meeting and helps maintain the focus on practice whilst enabling a questioning approach.

Driscoll (1994) agrees with this, but suggests that not all reflective practice is clinical supervision but potentially all good supervision is reflective practice. He also points out that clinical supervision is not only about reflecting on the big issues surrounding clinical practice but also on the seemingly insignificant and most ordinary of practice activities.

Driscoll's (2000) model of clinical supervision is probably the most widely known and used. It is in the form of reflective practice, but the essential difference is that it involves another person helping someone to reflect. It is cyclical in nature and is known as the WHAT? It contains three elements that are used for a supervisee to prepare for clinical supervision.

- WHAT? – a description of the event;
- So WHAT? – an analysis of the event;
- Now WHAT? – proposed actions following the event.

Driscoll (2000, p. 30) also lists a number of trigger questions, which are not dissimilar to those posed by Johns (2002) and Stephenson (1993, cited in Palmer *et al.*, 1994) but, in addition, he lists some skills and attributes required (of both supervisor and supervisee) for effective clinical supervision. They are:

- a willingness to learn from what happens in practice;
- being open enough to share elements of practice with other people;
- being motivated enough to replay aspects of clinical practice;
- having knowledge for clinical practice, which can emerge from within, as well as outside clinical practice;
- being aware of the conditions necessary for reflection to occur;
- a belief that it is possible to change as a practitioner;
- the ability to describe in detail before analysing practice problems;
- recognising the consequences of reflection;
- the ability to articulate what happens in practice;
- a belief that there is no end point about learning in practice;
- not being defensive about what other people notice about one's practice;
- being courageous enough to act on reflection;
- working out schemes to personally action what has been learned;
- being honest in describing clinical practice to others.

REFERENCES

Boud, D., Keogh, R. and Walkwe, D. (1985) *Reflection: Turning experience into learning.* London: Kogan Page

Brown, R. (1995) *Portfolio Development and Profiling For Nurses.* Central Health Studies, Dinton: Mark Allen Publishing

Burns, S. and Bulman, C. (2000) *The Reflective Practice in Nursing.* Oxford: Blackwell Science

Cottrell, S. (2003) *Skills for Success.* New York: Palgrave Macmillan

Cottrell, S. (2008) *The Study Skills Handbook* (4th edn). New York: Palgrave

Department of Health (1993) *A Vision for the Future: The nursing, midwifery and health visiting contribution to health and health care.* London: HMSO

Driscoll, J. (1994) 'Reflective practice for practice'. *Senior Nurse*, 14 (1): 47–50

Driscoll, J. (2000) *Practicing Clinical Supervision.* London: Ballière Tindall

Dewey, J. (1938) *Experience and Education.* Macmillan: New York, cited in: Jasper, M. (2006) *Professional Development, Reflection and Decision-Making*. Oxford: Blackwell

Fitzgerald, M. (2000) 'Clinical supervision and reflective practice', in Bulman, C. and Burns, S. (eds) *Reflective Practice In Nursing* (2nd edn, Ch. 5). Oxford: Blackwell Scientific

Gibbs, G. (1998) *Learning by Doing: A guide to teaching and learning methods*. London: Further Education Unit

Hurford, A. (2009) **www.nottingham.ac.uk/academicsupport/materials** (accessed March 2009)

Jasper, M. (2003) *Beginning Reflective Practice – Foundations in nursing and health care*. Cheltenham: Nelson Thornes

Jasper, M. (2006) *Professional Development, Reflection and Decision-Making*. Oxford: Blackwell

Johns, C. (2002) *Guided Reflection: Advancing practice*. Oxford: Blackwell

Kitson, K. (2005) **www.ibms.org** (accessed March 2009)

Moon, J. (2004) *A Handbook of Reflective and Experiential Learning*. London: Routledge

Nursing and Midwifery Council (2008a) *The Prep Handbook*. London: NMC

Nursing and Midwifery Council (2008b) *Clinical Supervision for Registered Nurses: Advice sheet*. London: NMC

Peate, I. (2006) *Becoming a Nurse in the 21st Century*. Chichester: John Wiley & Sons

Price, B. (2002) 'Effective learning no. 3: Reflective observations in practice'. *Nursing Standard*, 17 (9): S1–2

Royal College of Nursing (2002) *Clinical Supervision in the Workplace: Guidance for occupational health nurses*. London: RCN

Somerset Academy (2005) *Reflective Framework*. Somerset Academy

Stephenson, S. (1993) 'Reflection – A student perspective', cited in Palmer, A. Burns, S. and Bulman, C. (eds) (1994) *Reflective Practice In Nursing: The growth of the professional practitioner*. Oxford: Blackwell

Whitehead, E. and Mason, T. (2003) *Study Skills for Nurses*. London: Sage

Useful websites

www.nmc-uk.org/aArticle.aspx?ArticleID=330&Keyword=Persona l%20and%20professional%20and%20profile

Chapter 12

Study Skills, IT and Medicine Calculations

The aim of this chapter is to provide a brief overview of some of the key factors associated with study skills, using IT and medicine calculations.

Outcomes

On completion of this chapter you should be able to:

- identify and discuss some key study skills and the effective use of IT;
- display numeracy skills by accurately calculating medicine dosages and intravenous infusion rates.

STUDY SKILLS

The term 'study skills' can be defined as 'the skills you will need to become an effective and successful student' (**www.humanities.manchester. ac.uk**). Probably, if we are honest, most of us never really think about the skills required for studying – we just get on and do it. However, it is suggested that the more study skills and strategies you apply and practice, the more independent and confident you can become in any learning situation (**www.itscotland.org.uk**). It should also though be remembered that no two people study in exactly the same way, so what works for one person may well not work for another. The following section offers some widely recognised skills that you might like to try to see if they work for you.

Reading

When you start a nursing course you will have the same problem as every other student – how to get through the vast amount of reading you are required to do in order to complete the programme. There will not be enough time to read everything line by line so you will have to learn the skills that enable you to read efficiently and effectively within the time you have available. The following provides a brief overview of some of the main skills involved.

Environment

Think about the environment in which you are reading. It is most unlikely that you will be able to concentrate on reading and understanding if you are in an environment that is noisy and uncomfortable. Try to find a physical environment that is conducive for you to read in, for example by turning off the television or moving into another, quiet room or using a library. Other things you might consider include making sure the lighting is adequate, and that you are comfortably seated and working at a table if you are going to take notes. Try to work out which time of the day is best for you to study, and read at this time whenever possible. Try to avoid important reading if you are tired or if your eyes ache.

Styles or types of reading

Your style of reading should be chosen to suit the task. Styles or types of reading include the following.

Skimming

This is the technique you may use when you are going through a newspaper or magazine. The idea is that you read quickly to get the main points, and skip over the detail. It's also useful to skim when reading academic texts to:

- preview a passage before you read it in detail;
- refresh your understanding of a passage after you have read it in detail;
- decide if a book in the library or bookshop is right for you – to do this look at the title, author, synopsis (on back cover or front flap), contents page and date of publication for an indication of its relevance to your needs.

Scanning

Having decided on the potential usefulness of a book from your skim, you then need to confirm that it will indeed be useful to you for your studies. This involves a more in-depth examination or scanning of a text for specific information relevant to your task or topic area. This can include scanning:

- the synopsis on the back cover of the book;
- the introduction or preface of a book;
- the first or last paragraphs of chapters;
- the concluding chapter of a book.

Detailed reading

This is where you read sections and chapters in full and work to learn from the text.

Critical reading

Critical reading requires you to evaluate the information and arguments in the text. You need to distinguish fact from opinion, and look at arguments given for and against the various issues. This is also where, having read appropriately more than one text on a similar topic, you begin to identify and compare and contrast any bias, objectivity and perspective that they may have. Using such comparisons when writing an essay can help to contribute towards a more balanced and objective piece of work.

Reading skills

Active reading

When you are reading for your course you will need to make sure you are actively involved as much as possible with the text in order to help maintain your concentration and understanding.

Active reading can include a variety of techniques:

- **Underlining and highlighting** – pick out what you think are the most important parts of what you are reading. If you are a visual learner, you will find it helpful to use different colours to highlight different aspects of what you're reading. (NB: Do this with your own copy of texts or on photocopies, not with books or journals borrowed from the library, or from fellow students or lecturers.)

- **Note key words** – record the main headings as you read. Use one or two keywords for each point. When you do not want to mark the text, keep a folder of the notes you make while reading.

SQ3R method

One well-recognised model of active reading that incorporates some of these suggestions is the SQ3R method. The SQ3R method involves five steps that should, if followed, help you to get the most out of your reading. The five steps are:

1 survey;
2 question;
3 read;
4 recall/recite;
5 review.

- **S = Survey** – This first step helps you to gather information necessary to focus on the topic and helps orientate you to the author's purpose (what is he/she trying to get across to the reader?) and the main ideas in the text. Before reading, you need to survey the material. This can involve looking (glancing) at the title of the chapter, any boldface headings or subheadings, any visual aids to points for example, charts, maps, diagrams, and reading the chapter introduction and/or summary. Only a few minutes need be spent surveying the text to ease you into the reading.
- **Q = Question** – This step requires deliberate effort. The key here is to develop a questioning attitude as you are reading the chapter or text. This can be achieved by, for example, turning the title, headings and/or subheadings into questions (e.g. if the subheading is 'recording references' your question may be – 'why do I need to record references?'). It can also include looking at any questions that might be posed by the author through set activities or at the end of the chapter. Writing the questions down helps keeps you alert and helps focus your concentration on what you need to learn or get out of your reading.
- **R = Read** – For this step you need to actively read the material and try to answer any of the questions you have raised. Note down and answer questions in your own words as this will enable you to understand and comprehend more fully the text you are reading. Look for the main ideas and important details, notice italicised or bold words, study any visual aids and make sure you understand their meaning and/or relevance to the text. Reduce the speed of your reading for difficult passages of text, and stop and re-read parts that are not clear.

- **R = Recite or recall** – Keep challenging yourself to make sure you have an understanding of what you are reading by recitation and constant recall. After each section, stop and think back to your questions. See if you can answer them from memory. If not, take a look back at the text. Try to recall main headings, important issues and concepts in your own words and what graphs and charts indicate. Do these as often as you need, as this can help you learn and apply the knowledge to other areas.
- **R = Review** – The review is an assessment of what you have accomplished, not what you are going to do. When you have finished a chapter, article, etc., go back over the questions posed during your reading. See if you can still answer them. If not, look back and refresh your memory, even re-read if necessary. During review, it's a good time to go over notes you have taken to help clarify points you may have missed or don't understand. It can also be useful to make flash cards for important points or for those questions that you found difficult to answer. The best time to review is when you have just finished studying.

www.buzzin.net; www.education.exeter.ac.uk; www.arc.sbc.edu; www.studys.net; www.adprima.com

Taking notes

Note-taking is a skill that you will need to use many times as a student of nursing. Effective note-taking should have a purpose, should be well organised, and can be a time-saving skill. By making notes you actively process and interpret ideas and information; this aids concentration and understanding and should enable you to learn more. Notes can also play an important part in preparing and planning assignments and projects by helping you to identify main points and organise your ideas into a logical order. When preparing for an exam, notes can provide a concise record of information for you to revise from. There is no one 'correct' way to take notes. Everyone tends to develop their own way of taking notes, and very different approaches can be equally effective. The following are tips on how you might become an efficient and successful note-taker. These can apply equally to taking notes from a verbal presentation or from a written text.

Amount

The whole point of note-taking is to be able to summarise information in a different, shorter form to use later. Therefore, whichever strategy you use, it is important to realise you do not have to copy down everything you read or hear. If you do, note-taking will just become time-consuming, ineffective and a boring and passive way of learning.

Key words and phrases

When making notes listen/look out for key words and phrases such as 'the most important factor is'. In your notes key words and phrases should trigger your memory or lead on to other ideas/explanations, therefore they must be easy to find when you are reviewing your notes at a later date. This may be achieved by:

- underlining important points once, very important points twice;
- using capital letters;
- drawing boxes around the key words;
- drawing an asterisk (*) next to the main idea;
- going over the most important points with a highlighter pen;
- using different coloured inks for different themes or approaches.

Symbols and abbreviations

When you take notes, particularly in a lecture, seminar, etc., or even while on clinical placement, you will rarely have time to write in full sentences or, sometimes, even full words. It is therefore useful to develop your own set of symbols and abbreviations. Some of the more common ones, which you will probably already be aware of, include:

e.g.	for example
i.e.	that is
+	and/plus
=	equals
NB	note well
%	percentage
etc.	and so on
<	less than
>	greater than
\	therefore
a/c	account
no.	number
ref.	reference
vs	against/as opposed to
w/	with
w/o	without

Remember though – do keep a copy of any of your own abbreviations in the front of your notes file so that you can remember them at a later date.

Mind-mapping (spray diagram/spider diagram)

Mind maps offer a non-linear and diagrammatical way to organise key ideas from your lectures, seminars and reading. They also have the potential to present a large amount of information on one page and act as a summary for more detailed notes.

In a mind map the main topic or argument is placed at the centre of the page (Figure 1).

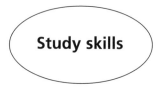

Figure 1 Main topic of a mind map

Ideas that relate to the main topic are then placed on branches that directly connect to the central topic (Figure 2).

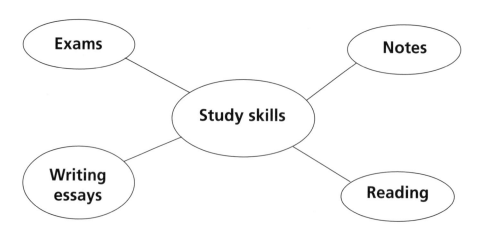

Figure 2 Main branches of a mind map

Each of these main ideas then develops its own branches of ideas (Figure 3).

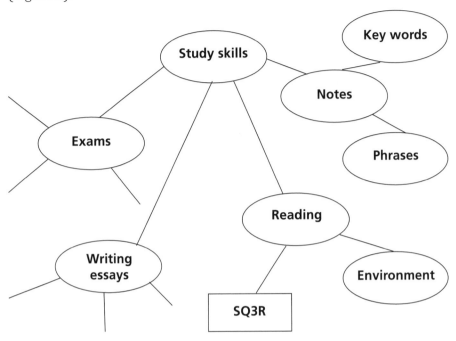

Figure 3 Further branches

As each theme is developed you add branch lines from each topic. Sometimes, it can also help to add colours and/or differently shaped boxes.

Once complete, when you have all your ideas down on paper, look for links between themes and indicate them with an arrow or chain. When using a mind map for an assignment, exam, etc., it can be useful to number each theme to show the order in which you are going to refer to them.

Handwriting, spelling and grammar

When you have completed a set of notes, check back and make sure that you can actually understand the notes you have made and that your handwriting has not become unreadable. Make any alterations while the topic is still fresh in your mind and/or when there are people around who can clarify what you should have written. As long as your meaning is clear don't worry about your spelling and grammar. At this stage it is better to focus on recording the information, so achieving perfection in spelling and grammar is not important – save this for your assignment or exam.

Plagiarism and paraphrasing

Plagiarism can become an issue, especially when taking notes from written texts. In order to avoid this, do not just copy down material verbatim from another source without putting it in quotation marks and noting its origin, i.e. always put the full reference and page number in the margin beside the quote. If you do not do this, you may well forget that these words are not your own. If you then include them as your own in an assignment, report, etc., you will have committed plagiarism. It is actually much better when taking notes to make sure you paraphrase (i.e. put a passage into your own words) wherever possible. If you do this at the note-taking stage, there can be no confusion later on.

Organise your notes

Although it seems to be common sense, it is surprising how many people do not organise effectively the notes they take during their course of study. It is important to have a good system for organising and storing your notes, as doing this well will save you a great deal of time when it comes to using them when preparing for an assignment or exam. As before, whatever system you decide to use or develop it should suit your personal needs. The following are some suggestions as to how your notes may be organised effectively.

- Use a separate file for each subject area.
- Use file dividers to separate major topics.
- Arrange notes under headings or questions.
- Number and label pages so that you can re-file them easily.
- Use one lecture note book per subject.
- Always leave a margin down one side of the page for future notes, references, comments, etc.

   www.jobs.ac.uk; www.humanities.manchester.ac.uk; www.trle.wiltscoll.ac.uk; www.english-zone.com

Writing essays

Writing essays is something that you will have to do on a regular basis in order to demonstrate your understanding and to show how much you have learnt about a topic in a well-structured written format. There is, once again, no single correct way to approach essay writing; each person needs to find what suits them best. The following section offers some tips to support or develop your approach.

Understanding the question

The basis of any essay should always begin from an understanding of what you are trying to achieve. It is therefore important that you should make sure that you know exactly what is required of you before you begin to research or to draft your essay. If you have been given a specific question, you need to begin by 'unpicking' the information it contains. This can be done by carefully examining the words of the question, looking for: the 'content words' that indicate the subject matter with which the essay should deal; the 'limiting words' that specify the particular aspect or aspects of the subject on which the essay should focus; and the 'instruction words' that tell you how to approach the topic. Therefore, essay questions usually contain one or more of the following key words that indicate what you are being asked to do.

- **Account for**: give reasons for, explain how something came about, clarify.
- **Assess**: decide the importance/value of something and give reasons.
- **Analyse**: examine in detail, consider the various parts of the whole and describe the interrelationship between them.
- **Comment on**: explain the importance of.
- **Compare**: examine the objects in question with a view to demonstrating their similarities.
- **Contrast**: examine the objects in question for the purpose of demonstrating differences or examine two or more opposing ideas or arguments to highlight their differences.
- **Define**: state precisely the meaning of something using examples – a simple statement is often not enough, the meaning needs to be explored in detail.
- **Discuss**: explain and give different views about something – this can include your own views as long as they are based on sound evidence (i.e. they are referenced).
- **Examine**: look at very carefully.
- **Explain**: make very clear why something is the way it is, or why it happens.
- **Evaluate**: examine the evidence and decide on the value of something, make a judgement about it, based on sound evidence.
- **Give an account of**: describe in detail how something happened.
- **Illustrate**: make something very clear, using evidence and examples.
- **Outline**: give a short description of the main points.
- **Justify**: support a particular idea, using evidence, and show why particular conclusions were made – include counter-arguments.
- **Show**: make clear, demonstrate evidence for.
- **Summarise**: outline the main points briefly.
- **To what extent**: discuss how accurate it is.

Essay planning

Once you have decided what is required, researched the topic and read through your notes, you should then make an essay plan. Time spent on essay planning is rarely time wasted as it provides an opportunity to identify the main themes, sections or areas and how all the various pieces of information fit together. An essay plan is also useful to take to a tutorial so that you can discuss with your tutor your ideas about completing the assignment. The plan should be written in a way that works for you personally, for example, as a mind map, linear notes or a set of boxes, etc.

Structure of an essay

The structure of the essay is important because it demonstrates that you are able to order your thoughts in a systematic, logical way and it provides a sense of direction through the essay. The accepted basic framework for any essay is:

- an introduction;
- a main body/text;
- a conclusion.

The introduction

The purpose of the introduction should be to set the context and direction of the essay. It should therefore:

- be clear that it is an introduction;
- if required, set the question topic against a wider background (set the context);
- identify and/or define any key terms;
- briefly summarise the overall theme of the essay, indicating the main points to be made and, possibly, the order in which they are to be presented – that is, explain what the essay is going to do.

Main body/text

The main body of the text is where the main ideas or arguments are developed. Depending on the length of the essay, it will contain several sections, each divided into paragraphs. The paragraphs should be logically linked as you develop the themes or ideas. In the main body you should:

- present key points clearly;

- present ideas or arguments backed up by evidence from your reading;
- accurately cite quotations and references to other works;
- label any diagrams, figures or tables correctly.

Conclusion

The conclusion should follow logically from, and be based on, what you have presented in the main body of your essay as it brings together the main ideas explored. This can be achieved by:

- briefly summarising the main ideas and arguments;
- linking back to the title/topic, showing how you have answered the question and drawn a relevant conclusion;
- making clear why conclusions reached are important or significant;
- not including any new ideas.

Referencing

Referencing is the standardised method of acknowledging sources of information. When writing an essay, report or dissertation, it is usual to make reference (i.e. to identify the place where the original citation can be found) to the sources that you used, referred to, or took quotes from. These references might be from, for example, a journal, newspaper articles, books or book chapters, government reports, internet publications. When you refer to, or directly quote from, someone else's work you must refer to the author/editor both in the text and in a reference list or bibliography at the end of your work. Citing accurate references in academic work is important for the following reasons.

- To give credit to other authors' concepts and ideas.
- To provide evidence of the extent of your reading.
- To allow a reader to locate the cited references easily.
- It is vital to avoid being accused of plagiarism.

Plagiarism can be defined as: 'taking and using another person's thoughts, inventions and writings as one's own' (*Oxford English Dictionary*, 1988, p. 616). This is potentially a serious offence in an academic environment, but can be easily avoided by acknowledging all sources of information. Failure to do this could result in work being downgraded or even unmarked. The reference list should contain details of all the sources you have mentioned in your essay. A bibliography contains sources you have consulted but not mentioned in your essay. You may be asked for just a reference list or you may be asked for both references and a bibliography. You need to check your assignment guidelines to see what is required.

There are many systems for the citation of references, and you should follow the system that will be identified in your course handbook or assessment guidelines. The most commonly used systems in the UK are the Harvard system and the Vancouver system.

Harvard system

The Harvard system cites the author's surname and year of publication in the text, e.g. (Jones, 2004), and provides a reference list (of any text citations), in alphabetical order by author at the end of the assignment. It is here that additional details are noted, such as surname and initials, the title of the article, book or chapter, place of publication and the publisher.

Vancouver system

In the Vancouver system, a number is assigned to each reference as it is used. Even if the author is named in the text, a number must still be used. The original number assigned to the reference is used each time that reference is cited in the text. The first reference cited will be numbered 1 in the text, and the second reference cited will be numbered 2, and so on. If a reference cited number 1 is used again later in the text, it should be cited using the number 1 again. References are listed in numerical order in a reference list/bibliography at the end of the essay.

A few final points about essays

Style of writing

Precision of language is very important. Ensure that your writing style:

- utilises complete, straightforward sentences that are varied, not too simple or too convoluted (complex sentences do not necessarily signify complex thought), and also avoids writing in note form;
- avoids using slang and colloquialisms;
- only quote relevant material and does not overuse quotes (much better to interpret information in your own words);
- does not use inappropriate analogies;
- does not adopt a subjective or emotive tone;
- does not make assertions or sweeping statements without supporting evidence or argument;
- is not repetitive.

Paragraphs

There should be one main theme per paragraph and you should signal the natural breaks in your argument when the focus of attention shifts.

Excessively long paragraphs should be avoided and where possible, the first sentence of each paragraph should link in some way to the previous paragraph. This allows for the flow or continuity of argument, which is a very important quality in essays.

Link words

Link words are words that provide 'signposts' along the way, which help identify connections and relationships between key ideas. They include:

- words that lead the reader forwards, such as 'again', 'furthermore', 'finally';
- words that make the reader stop and compare, such as 'however', 'although', 'nonetheless';
- words that develop and summarise, such as 'obviously', 'therefore', 'in conclusion'.

Length

The length of any assignment will be identified in the assignment guidelines. It is important that you are as close to your word limit as possible, as most universities or colleges will probably have clearly identified mark penalties if the word count of an assignment is at least 10 per cent over or under the stated amount for that piece of work. Usually it will be requested that you record your word count at the end of the assignment and, again, failure to do so might result in the loss of some marks.

Proofread

The final preparation of the essay for submission is important. This includes carefully proofreading your essay, or asking a friend or relative to do this for you. Even better is getting someone to read your work back to you. Notice any faults of grammar and make sure you correct them before submitting the work. Spelling errors can sometimes be more difficult to detect, simply because you do not know the way in which a particular word is spelt. Nevertheless, you should try to correct as many spelling errors as possible. Most word-processing packages now include spelling and grammar checks – use both but don't rely on them completely as some words may be spelt correctly but used in the wrong context like, for example, 'write' and 'right'.

Presentation

Print out your work in hard copy, preferably using double spacing or 1.5 line spacing when word-processing, and include wide margins (both make the text far easier to read and comment upon).

NB: Don't forget to keep at least one copy of your assignment; they can occasionally get lost in the system.

> **www.data.bolton.ac.uk; www.staffs.ac.uk; www.shef.ac.uk; www.2.napier.ac.uk; www.lib.gla.ac.uk**

Using information technology (IT)

Over the past decade information technology has significantly changed the way ideas and information are recorded and communicated in all areas of life, including the study (and practice) of nursing. According to Northedge (2007, pp. 51–52), computers help with studies in several different ways, including:

- researching online;
- making notes;
- managing your studies – helping to organise and keep track of studies;
- word-processing;
- working with numbers and charts – computer software can be perfect for creating tables, charts and graphs;
- storing information;
- talking online;
- e-learning.

It is beyond the scope of this section to explore all of the above in any depth. However, a few tips are offered for researching online and the issue of e-learning will be explored a little further.

Researching online

Some general tips include the following.

Narrow your research topic

The internet allows access to so much information that you can easily be overwhelmed so, before you start your search, think about what you're looking for and, if possible, formulate some very specific questions to direct and limit your search. Try not to use broad or general terms – rather use terms that are more specific to the topic you are researching. You can also sometimes narrow your search by looking at sites that you may have previously used and that are relevant to your topic.

Boolean operators

Boolean operators are words that allow you to combine search terms and can be utilised in most search engines. They are 'and', 'or' and 'not'.

- **and** – narrows the search and retrieves sites/records containing all the words it separates. For example, entering 'values AND ethics' would instruct the search engine to find web pages that contain both words, 'values' and 'ethics'.
- **or** – broadens the search and retrieves sites/records containing any of the words it separates. For example, entering 'values OR ethics' would cause the search engine to look for web pages that contain either the word 'values' or the word 'ethics', but not necessarily both words. You need to be mindful that this could result in the return of thousands or even millions of sites. 'Or' is most useful when the same term may appear in two different ways like, for example, using 'evidence-based practice OR EBP' to find information about evidence-based practice.
- **not** – narrows the search and retrieves sites that do not contain the term following the 'not' – i.e. it finds the first word but not the second. This limitation is helpful when you know your search term is likely to appear with another term that does not interest you, for example, 'toddler NOT baby'.

Exact phrases

If you want your search engine to search for an exact phrase, put quotation marks around the phrase.

Include appropriate alternative or synonymous terms

Scan the titles and abstracts of the sites/records you find for other possible keywords or synonyms you may not have thought of using. For example, a search on the common name 'St John's wort' finds records which include the Latin name *hypericum* and the extract name 'hypericin'. A good revised search strategy would therefore be: 'St John's wort OR hypericum OR hypericin'.

Know your subject directories and search engines

Search engines (for example, Google, Yahoo and AltaVista) can differ considerably in the way they work, how much of the internet they search, and the kind of results you can expect to get from them. Spending some time learning what each search engine will do and how best to use it can help you avoid a lot of frustration and wasted time later. There are a great many good academic resources available on the internet, including hundreds of online journals and sites set up by universities and scholarly or nursing organisations. The following are some core bibliographic e–resources.

- The BNI (British Nursing Index) provides reference to journals and articles, some conference papers and major reports on aspects of education and nursing from the UK and some English-language international publications.
- CINAHL (Cumulative Index to Nursing and Allied Health Literature) has international coverage and indexes over 1600 nursing and allied health journals.
- CRD (Centre for Reviews and Dissemination) enables the search of the Database of Abstracts of Reviews of Effects (DARE), the NHS Economic Evaluation Database (NHS EED) and the Health Technology Assessment database (HTA).
- The Cochrane Library is designed to provide evidence to inform health care decision-making.
- MEDLINE (Medical Literature Analysis and Retrieval System Online), ASSIA (Applied Social Science Index and Abstracts), IBSS (International Bibliography of the Social Sciences).

Evaluate the information

If you are not using recognised academic resources such as those above, you need to remember that anyone can put anything they want to on a website; there is no review or screening process, and there are no agreed-upon standard ways of identifying subjects and creating cross-references. Therefore, you must always ensure that you think critically about the information you have found on the internet. Some of the questions you should be asking yourself are:

- who is the author?
- who is sponsoring the website?
- what is the audience level?
- is the information current and up to date?
- is the content reliable and accurate?

Remember that if you decide to use the information, you are responsible for ensuring that it is reliable and accurate. (See Chapter 8 on 'Evidence-based practice' for further hints on how to review articles.)

Keep a detailed record of sites you visit and the sites you use

Doing research on the internet inevitably means visiting some sites that are useful and many that are not. Keeping a record of useful websites is good practice so that you can revisit them at a later date. Also, if using the information in an essay, etc., you can more easily and accurately acknowledge the source of that information. Using the browser's history function for this is not really good practice as it will retain all the web addresses or URLs of the sites you visit, good or bad. Also, if you are using a computer at your place of study the memory in the history file will be erased at the end of your session. It is much better to either note down (accurately) on paper or bookmark the sites you've found useful, so that you will have a permanent record.

Double-check all URLs that you put in your paper

It is easy to make mistakes with complicated internet addresses and typing errors will invalidate your references. If you type them into the location box of your browser you will be able to check that you have the correct address because it will take you to the correct site.

Don't rely exclusively on internet resources

Generally speaking you will be expected to make use of both internet and library resources. Cross-checking information from the internet against information from the library can be a good way to make sure that the internet material is reliable and authoritative.

> **www.lsa.ac.uk; owl.english.purdue.edu; www.utm.utoronto.ca; www.unmec.edu; www.csa.com**
>
> (Northedge, 2007)

Electronic learning (e-learning)

E-learning is a unifying term used to describe the learning and delivery of a training or education programme using a computer or electronic device (for example, a mobile phone). Over the past decade its use has been steadily increasing within nursing programmes both at pre- and post-registration levels. Some other terms frequently interchanged with 'e-learning' include:

- online learning;
- online education;
- distance education;
- distance learning;
- technology-based training;
- web-based training;
- computer-based training (generally thought of as learning from a CD-ROM).

Types of e-learning

E-learning comes in many variations and is often a combination of two or more of the following:

- purely online – no face-to-face meetings;
- blended learning – combination of online and face-to-face;
- synchronous – live interaction between tutor and students – students log in at a specific time and for a specified duration;
- asynchronous – students learn through internet-based, network-based or stored disk-based modules – interaction with others includes via e.mail, online discussion groups and online bulletin boards;
- teacher-led group;
- self-study;
- web-based study;
- computer-based (CD-ROM) study;
- video/audio tape.

Features and benefits of e-learning

Wherever you look in the literature it is clear that the use of e-learning can demonstrate significant benefits. These benefits are that:

- learning is self-paced and provides the learner with a chance to speed up or slow down as necessary;
- learning is self-directed, thus allowing a learner to choose content and tools appropriate to their differing interests, needs, and skill levels;
- range and course availability can be significantly increased;
- it allows for multiple learning styles using a variety of delivery methods geared to different learners;
- it tends to be more learner-centred;
- accessibility is anytime and anywhere;
- online learning does not require physical attendance at a particular place and time;
- it can encourage greater student interaction and collaboration;
- it can encourage greater student/teacher contact;
- it enhances computer and internet skills;
- it provides global opportunities for learning.

  www.direct.gov.uk; www.worldwidelearn.com; www.tech-faq.com; www.agelesslearner.com

> **Further reading**
>
> There is a considerable amount of information on the internet regarding study skills. You should be able to start your search using a general search engine such as **www.google.co.uk** and the websites referred to in this chapter.
>
> Lloyd, M. and Murphy, P. (2008) *Essential Study Skills for Health and Social Care*. Exeter: Reflect Press, is highly recommended as a guide for anyone with a serious interest in the long-term development of their learning and study skills.

MEDICINE CALCULATIONS

'Mathematical accuracy is a matter of life and death in clinical nursing' (Keighley, 1984, cited in Cheung, 1986) is an old reference, but certainly one that is still relevant. Drug errors account for 25 per cent of all litigation claims to the NHS (Wright, 2005) and improving the drug calculation skills of nurses is one strategy identified by the Department of Health to try to reduce this number by 40 per cent (Department of Health, 2004). The Department of Health (2004) also states that medication errors are costing the NHS between £200 and £400 million per year. The guidelines for administration of medicines (NMC, 2008, p. 28) state:

> Some drug administrations can require complex calculations to ensure that the correct volume or quantity of medication is administered. In these situations, it is good practice for a second practitioner (a registered professional) to check the calculation independently in order to minimise the risk of error. The use of calculators to determine the volume or quantity of medication should not act as a substitute for arithmetical knowledge and skill.

Drug dosages and infusion rates

To calculate drug dosages and intravenous infusion rates, competence in the use of both fractions and decimals is required. The formulae suggested here are calculated in fractions, while the end result must be in decimals for administration. However, when calculating drugs dosages a certain amount of logic is also required – nurses should be encouraged to predict mentally what the answer might be. Consider the following example:

The dose ordered is chlorphenamine 3 mg. The stock dose is 2 mg in 5 ml. Is the answer going to be greater or less than 5 ml?

Fractions

1. Simplifying or cancelling down fractions.

To simplify a fraction, divide the top and bottom figures by a common denominator (a number that will go into both). For example:

$$\frac{25}{75} = \frac{1}{3} \qquad \text{Both figures have been divided by 25}$$

This calculation may be done in more than one step:

e.g. $\frac{25}{75}$ (both divided by 5) $= \frac{5}{15}$ (both divided by 5) $= \frac{1}{3}$

Activity

Simplify the following fractions:

1a. $\frac{12}{28}$ b. $\frac{8}{12}$ c. $\frac{75}{150}$ d. $\frac{100}{250}$

e. $\frac{1600}{8000}$ f. $\frac{120}{150}$ g. $\frac{1250}{1600}$ h. $\frac{18}{3}$

Answers to all the activities are at the end of the chapter.

---

2. Changing fractions to decimals.

To change a fraction into a decimal, divide the top number by the bottom number:

e.g. $\frac{1}{4}$ becomes $4\overline{)1.00}$ .25

Activity

Change the following to decimals:

2a. $\dfrac{1}{5}$ **b.** $\dfrac{1}{2}$ **c.** $\dfrac{1}{10}$

To simplify larger numbers like, for example $\dfrac{800}{1600}$

it is easier to divide the top and bottom figures by 100 (i.e. delete the zeros), leaving

$$\frac{8}{16} = \frac{1}{2}$$

Decimals

Drugs are usually administered in:

* grams (g);
* milligrams (mg);
* micrograms (µg);
* millilitres (ml).

1 kilogram (kg)	=	1000 grams
1 gram (g)	=	1000 milligrams
1 milligram (mg)	=	1000 micrograms (µg)
1 litre (l)	=	1000 millilitres (ml)

To carry out drug calculations it may be necessary to convert one unit to another. For example, if the strength of the dose you have is in milligrams, the end calculation must also be in milligrams. Thus, you would first have to convert the dose required to milligrams. Remember that these units are SI units and therefore always increase or decease in multiples of 1000.

1. The multiplication of decimals.

This can be done by simply moving the decimal point.

To multiply by	Move the decimal point
10	1 place to the right
100	2 places to the right
1000	3 places to the right

For example:

2.0 × 1000 = 2000	Decimal point moved 3 places to the right
1.3 × 100 = 130	Decimal point moved 2 places to the right
0.6 × 10 = 6	Decimal point moved 1 place to the right

Activity

Try the following:

2d. 0.075 × 10   **e.** 0.003 × 100   **f.** 0.01 × 1000

g. 0.2 × 1000   **h.** 0.0505 × 100   **i.** 7.7 × 1000

2. The division of decimals.

For division of decimals move the point the other way – to the left.

To divide by:	Move the decimal point
10	1 place to the left
100	2 places to the left
1000	3 places to the left

For example:

37.8 ÷ 10	= 3.78	Decimal point moved 1 place to the left
37.8 ÷ 100	= 0.378	Decimal point moved 2 places to the left
37.8 ÷ 1000	= 0.0378	Decimal point moved 3 places to the left

---

Drug calculations formula

$$\frac{\text{what you want}}{\text{what you've got}} \quad \times \quad \frac{\text{what it's in}}{1}$$

For example:

You have 80 mg in 10 ml – you want 200 mg

$$\frac{200}{80} \quad \times \quad \frac{10}{1} \quad = \quad 25 \text{ ml}$$

As previously stated it is essential that the units are the same in the calculation so that, for example, you have 4 g in 250 ml and you require 800 mg, therefore you need to convert the 4 g to milligrams first before applying the formula:

$$\frac{800}{4000} \quad \times \quad \frac{250}{1} \quad = \quad 50 \text{ ml}$$

Activity

Complete these drug calculations:	
Dose ordered	**Stock amp/soln**
3a. Ampicillin 350 mg	500 mg in 100 ml
3b. Pethidine 125 mg	100 mg in 1 ml
3c. Phenobarbitone 140 mg	200 mg in 1 ml
3d. Heparin 1250 units	25000 units in 1 ml
3e. Potassium chloride 16 mmol	26 mmol in 10 ml
3f. Digoxin 150 µg	55 µg in 2 ml
3g. Scopolamine 0.3 mg	0.4 mg in 1 ml
3h. Methicillin 1750 mg	1 g in 2.5 ml

Timing the infusion

Intravenous fluids should be prescribed in millilitres, but if they are prescribed in litres this must be converted to millilitres before any calculation can take place.

British Standard adult infusion sets give 15, 20 or 60 drops per ml.

Blood sets	=	15 drops per ml (when blood is transfused)
Solution sets	=	20 drops per ml
Burette sets	=	60 drops per ml

To calculate the drops per minute:

$$\frac{\text{Volume of fluid to be infused}}{\text{Hours}} \times \frac{\text{Number of drops per ml of giving set}}{60 \text{ (minutes)}}$$

e.g. 500 ml of normal saline to be infused over 4 hours

$$\frac{500}{4} \times \frac{20}{60} = 41 \text{ drops per minute}$$

Activity

Complete the following calculations:

4. Using a standard 20 drops per ml infusion set, calculate the number of drops per minute to infuse the following:

   a. 300 ml over 4 hours b. 145 ml over 1 hour

   c. 500 ml over 2.5 hours d. 800 ml over 6 hours

   e. 300 ml over 3 hours

5. Using a blood administration set (15 drops per ml), calculate the following in drops per minute:

a. 150 ml over 2 hours   **b.** 375 ml over 6 hours

c. 225 ml over 3 hours   **d.** 125 ml over 2 hours

e. 165 ml over 2.5 hours

6. Using a paediatric burette set (60 drops per ml), calculate the following drip rates to infuse:

a. 320 ml over 4 hours   **b.** 125 ml over 1 hour

c. 250 ml over 4 hours   **d.** 150 ml over 1 hour

e. 50 ml over 30 minutes

DRUG ABBREVIATIONS

Abbreviation	English
ac	before meals
ad lib	freely
alte die	alternate days
am	morning
bid/bd	twice a day
c	with
cap	capsule
ext	external use
gtt	drops
m	send
mg	milligrams
ml	millilitres
nocte	at night
od	once a day
o	oral/by mouth
pc	after meals
pm	evening
po	by mouth/oral

prn	as needed/required
qds	four times a day
s	without
sig ut dict	take as directed
stat	at once/straight away
tab	tablet
tds	three times a day
top	apply topically to body

Further reading

Davison, N. (2008) *Numeracy, Clinical Calculations and Basic Statistics: A textbook for health care students.* Exeter: Reflect Press, is a useful guide for nursing students who want to practise and develop their clinical calculation skills.

REFERENCES

Cheung, P. (1986) 'Learning your tables'. *Nursing Times*, 84 (40): 40–41

Department of Health (2004) *Building a Safer NHS for Patients: Improving Medication Safety*. London: Department of Health

Northedge, A. (2007) *The Good Study Guide*. Milton Keynes: Open University Press

Nursing and Midwifery Council (2008) *Standards for Medicine Management* (full content). London: NMC

Oxford English Dictionary (1988) *The Oxford English Dictionary*. Oxford: Oxford University Press

Wright, K. (2005) 'An exploration into the most effective way to teach drug calculation skills to nursing students'. *Nurse Education Today*, 25: 430–436

Useful websites

hedc.otago.ac.nz/hedc/sld/Study-Guides-and-Resources/Essay-Writing.html (accessed 12/4/09)

www2.napier.ac.uk/getready/writing_presenting/essays.html (accessed 12/4/09)

www.new2teaching.org.uk/tzone/Students/essays/default.asp (accessed 12/4/09) www.itscotland.org.uk/studyskills/about/index.asp (accessed 12/4/09)

www.humanities.manchester.ac.uk/studyskills/general (accessed 12/4/09)

www.adprima.com/studyout.htm (accessed 12/4/09)

www.buzzin.net/revision_tips/skills/rd-01.htm (accessed 12/4/09)

www.education.exeter.ac.uk/dll/studyskills/reading_skills.htm (accessed 12/4/09)

www.arc.sbc.edu/sq3r.html (accessed 12/4/09)

www.studys.net/texred2.htm (accessed 12/4/09)

www.wiltscoll.ac.uk/ap/Docs/Files/3/8/3/default.htm (accessed 12/4/09)

www.english-zone.com/study/symbols.htm (accessed 12/4/09)

www.jobs.ac.uk/career/tips/1006/Top_ten_tips_on_notetaking (accessed 12/4/09)

www.shef.ac.uk/scharr/ir/refman/manref/5majref.htm (accessed 12/4/09)

www.lib.gla.ac.uk/researchskills/citationstyle.shtml (accessed 12/4/09)

www.staffs.ac.uk/unisevices/infoservices/library/find/references/index.php (accessed 12/4/09)

www.data.boulton.ac/learning/helpguides/studyskills/essays.pdf (accessed 12/4/09)

www.lsa.ac.uk/004_health/nursing/nur_db.htm (accessed 12/4/09)

owl.english.purdue.edu/internet/search/index.html (accessed 12/4/09)

www.utm.utoronto.ca/library/instruction/researchinternet.html (accessed 12/4/09)

www.unmec.edu/library/educationdatabase/litstrat.html (accessed 12/4/09)

www.csa.com/help/search_Tools/boolean_operators.html (accessed 12/4/09)

www.direct.gov.uk/en/EducationAndLearning/AdultLearning/LearningOutsideTheClassroom/DG_4016860 (accessed 12/4/09)

www.worldwidelearn.com/learning-essentials/index.html (accessed 12/4/09)

www.tech-faq.com/e-/earning.shtml (accessed 12/4/09)

www.agelesslearner.com/intros/elearning.html (accessed 12/4/09)

Drug calculation answers

1a	$\frac{3}{7}$	1b	$\frac{2}{3}$	1c	$\frac{1}{2}$	1d	$\frac{2}{5}$
1e	$\frac{1}{5}$	1f	$\frac{4}{5}$	1g	$\frac{25}{32}$	1h	6
2a	0.2	2b	0.5	2c	0.1		
2d	0.75	2e	0.3	2f	10	2g	200
2h	5.05	2i	7700				
3a	70 ml	3b	1.25 ml	3c	0.7 ml	3d	0.05 ml
3e	6.15 ml	3f	5.45 ml	3g	0.75 ml	4h	4.38 ml

Infusion rate answers

4a	25	4b	48.3	4c	66.6	4d	44.4
4e	33.3						
5a	18.75	5b	15.6	5c	18.75	5d	15.6
5e	16.5						
6a	80	6b	125	6c	62.5	6d	150
6e	100						

Index

Added to a page number 'f' denotes a figure